Co...
and...

Nov...
to treat eac... ...TH ROOKLEDGE
Hertfordshire

I found the ...ook very help...u... ...ines all my
life and ha... been inspired to ... ...y
migraines ...nd headaches. I fe... ...NE ZALESKI
London

I have enjoyed reading through this very comprehensive book. The style is
excellent, based on the types of questions we are regularly asked.

ANN TURNER
Director, Migraine Action Association

It is comprehensive and the information is detailed and clear.

WENDY THOMAS
Chief Executive, The Migraine Trust

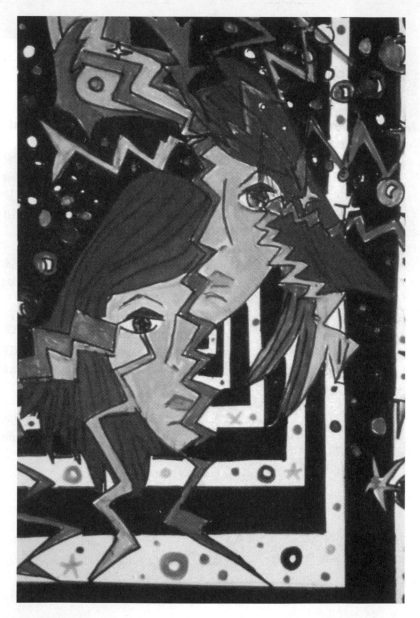

Frontispiece From the Migraine Art collection, reproduced by kind permission of the Migraine Action Association and Boehringer Ingelheim

Migraine
and other Headaches
Answers at your fingertips

Manuela Fontebasso

*General Practitioner and GP with Special Interest in Headache
Senior Honorary Clinical Tutor, Hull York Medical School*

CLASS PUBLISHING · LONDON

First published 2007

The author and publishers welcome feedback from the users of this book.
Please contact the publishers.

Class Publishing, Barb House, Barb Mews, London W6 7PA, UK
Telephone: 020 7371 2119 / Fax: 020 7371 2878 [International +4420]
email: post@class.co.uk / website: www.class.co.uk

The information presented in this book is accurate and current to the best
of the author's knowledge. The author and publisher, however, make no
guarantee as to, and assume no responsibility for, the correctness, sufficiency
or completeness of such information or recommendation. The reader is
advised to consult a doctor regarding all aspects of individual health care.

A CIP catalogue record for this book is available from the British Library

ISBN 10: 1 85959 149 3

ISBN 13: 978 1 85959 149 9

10 9 8 7 6 5 4 3 2 1

Edited by Lillian Clark

Designed and typeset by Martin Bristow

Artwork by David Woodroffe

Cartoons by Jane Taylor

Printed and bound in Finland by WS Bookwell, Juva

Contents

About the author

Manuela Fontebasso has been involved in headache since 1997 and is now a GP with Special Interest in Headache. She is also lead clinician for the headache clinic in the Department of Neuroscience at York Hospital and is Honorary Senior Clinical Tutor teaching first- and second-year medical students at the Hull York Medical School.

Manuela is a member of the British Association for the Study of Headache (BASH) and is on the BASH council with a special interest in education. She is also a member of the American Headache Society, of Migraine in Primary Care Advisors (MIPCA), a committee member of HEADACHE UK and is Honorary Medical Adviser to the Migraine Action Association.

She writes a range of articles for health-care journals and has lectured and run workshops for a wide range of health-care professionals as well as patient groups. She has given radio, television and newspaper interviews to raise the profile of headache in the general population.

Acknowledgements

First I thank all the team at Class Publishing, as, without their gentle but firm nurturing, I really would have given up on this project a long time ago.

I thank all those people I have met in the headache field who have inspired me, supported me and encouraged me over the years, especially Jill Murphy, my specialist nurse, who has read this book in its various drafts and offered helpful feedback along the way.

I also thank Peter Harrison who, as a great friend, work colleague and mentor, has always encouraged me to pursue my dreams when it came to taking up a new challenge or saying 'yes' to a new project. Peter, thank you for being such a kind and generous friend over the years, and I hope you and Di continue to thrive during your retirement.

The Frontispiece and Plates – examples of artwork by people who suffer from migraine – are from the Migraine Art collection and are reproduced by kind permission of the Migraine Action Association and Boehringer Ingelheim.

This book is dedicated to my family and friends but especially to my parents, whose support has allowed me to do all the things I have wanted to do and who have always been there to help when I have needed them. Thank you.

Foreword

Migraine and other Headaches: Answers at your fingertips has much to offer both the newly diagnosed migraine patient and the more knowledgeable sufferer of long experience.

Migraine is a complex neurological condition which affects people in many different ways. The combination of symptoms, triggers, treatments and effects on quality of life are peculiar to each individual. Migraine can also vary from attack to attack and may evolve throughout the lifetime of the sufferer. Each patient has to find their own personal solution to enable them to feel in control of *their* migraine. This can be like fitting together a jigsaw from a myriad different pieces, many of which are not required. It is therefore small wonder that patients seldom obtain the answers to all of their many questions during an average 7–10 minute consultation with their GP.

This excellent book provides the answers to many of those questions in a simple, straightforward but unpatronising manner. Its format makes it easy for readers to quickly find the information they are seeking, and the wide variety of questions and extensive cross-referencing lead easily to related information and answers to any subsequent questions they may have.

People are now encouraged to take greater responsibility for their own health care and participate in shared decision-making on treatment options. This book provides understandable information to enable them to do these things effectively.

Ann Turner
Director
Migraine Action Association

Foreword

Dr Manuela Fontebasso has written a very informative book for those who live with migraine and headache. It is clear that, as a GP with a special interest in headache, Dr Fontebasso has written from the front line of primary care and she has addressed hundreds of real-life issues that her patients bring to her on a daily basis. She has made her extensive and exhaustive knowledge of the subject available in accessible language, and her commitment to the support of people who live with disabling headaches shines through every page.

This book contains much that will empower the proactive migraineur, including over-the-counter options at the pharmacy, complementary therapies and lifestyle issues.

At The Migraine Trust we recognise how important it is for people to understand their headache condition, and this book fulfils a real need.

We highly recommend it to the lay person who wants to know more about their migraines and to the clinician who understands the importance of the informed patient.

Wendy Thomas
Chief Executive
The Migraine Trust

1 | Introduction

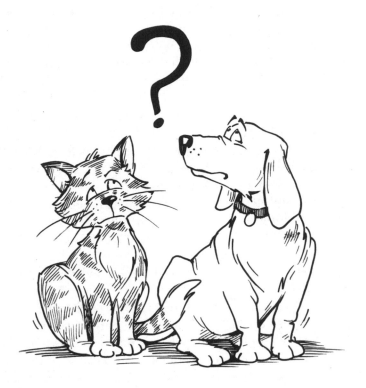

Writing this book has been quite a journey – an enjoyable one, sometimes a challenging one and hopefully a rewarding one. At least it will be rewarding if you read it and find something, even if it is only one thing, that you find to be helpful or useful or gives you one of those 'eureka' moments.

I have been a GP for over 20 years and been interested in headache in all its shapes and forms for nearly a decade. As a GP, every consultation is different, every person is an individual, every story is unique. As a headache specialist, every person I see has a story to tell and that story is theirs and theirs alone. The only way to understand that story is to listen to what that person has to say, to know every aspect of their experience and every last detail.

Being able to diagnose a problem or to understand a symptom or series of symptoms is all about the story – taking the history. Time is a precious commodity but there is no substitute for making the time to hear the story in the patient's own words. As a GP, a typical consultation lasts 10 minutes, occasionally longer; as a headache specialist, my first consultation lasts 40 minutes, often longer. As a GP, I may know the patient well; as a headache specialist, I am meeting that person for the first time.

Getting the information I need to make a diagnosis means I have to ask the right questions and listen carefully to the answers. I cannot make assumptions about what words and phrases mean: I have to be absolutely certain. Identifying each headache is about recognising a particular combination of symptoms and fitting them together to make a diagnosis. There are many different headaches, and this book tries to deal with the most common. It would be impossible to consider them all, and I am sorry if I have not included the one that you wanted to find out about.

I have departed from the usual format when reflecting on specialist services in Chapter 10, and the reasons for doing that were complex. I felt very strongly that the main purpose of this book was to empower you to find out as much as possible about your headache. By outlining the sorts of questions I ask and explaining why I ask them, I hope that you will be able to think a little bit more about your headache and all the associated symptoms and features before seeking advice from your GP. It is not always easy to find a health-care professional who is sympathetic to the headache sufferer, let alone having the depth of knowledge needed to offer the right advice on how to treat it.

Once a diagnosis has been made, it is time to think about what to do about it. In the same way that every person is different, so every headache is different. Managing headache is not just about taking pills or potions; it is about taking positive steps. As a headache specialist, I tend to adopt a fairly pragmatic approach and to encourage every patient I see to consider all the possible diet and lifestyle changes first and foremost. The ideas and suggestions offered in this book are based on the experience that I have gained as well as the evidence from scientific research.

Treating headache means using the right drug for the right headache. It means taking that drug at the right time and at the right dose. Every person is different, every headache is different and every treatment is different. There is a difference between the *acute treatment* of a headache (getting rid of the headache when it is there) and the *preventative treatment* of that headache (stopping the headache from happening in the first place). Ideas, experiences and expectations vary from person to person; the challenge is to translate those ideas, experiences and expectations into a reality. In this book I have tried to use the questions I have been asked by the patients I have seen in a clear and practical guide through the trials and pitfalls of all the options possible when treating migraine and all those other headaches.

Although it is important for you to feel in control of your migraine, it is not always practical or realistic to improve your headache on your own. Help, support and assistance are available – you just have to remember to ask for it or seek it out. Help can come from many different people and places, and sometimes it can be found only with a leap of faith. You do not have to do the difficult things on your own, though; things can change. Sometimes they just don't change quickly enough for you but patience can and does have its own reward.

I have dedicated a whole chapter to medication overuse headache (MOH) because it is a condition that is very difficult to treat but in its own way very rewarding to manage. In writing this particular chapter I have drawn widely on both the published scientific and research evidence and my experience over the last decade. MOH is a very common headache type; facilitating and empowering change is a task that needs a committed and motivated headache sufferer combined with the support of their friends, family and work colleagues, as well as their specialist, the specialist nurse and the GP.

Children get headaches, too. Children of parents who get headache are often more likely to get headache as well. Diagnosing headache in children can be just as challenging as making the diagnosis in an adult. Treating headache in children involves the same sorts of steps and decisions as those taken by adults but the person making the decisions is not always the person with the headache.

Women are more likely to get migraine than men, so it is not surprising that hormones feature in any book on headaches and, specifically, migraine. The answers offered are in part based on the 'evidence' but also on experience. It is another area where trial and error is often the only way forward.

I hope that, as you dip into and out of parts of this book, you find the answers to some, if not all, of your questions. There may be times when the answers are what you want to hear, and sometimes the answers may seem unwelcome. Improving headache symptoms is often about making change and ensuring that the changes made are positive rather than negative – they are about things you can do to make a difference not things you can't.

You need to understand what your headache is, know the best way to treat it, be involved in all areas of decision-making and, above all, take control so that you can feel in control and finally be in control.

2 | What is migraine?

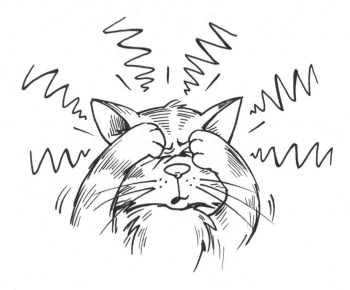

Migraine is a condition that can affect anyone at any time. Some people are more likely to experience migraine attacks than others but, if the right mix of conditions come together, almost anyone can experience a migraine.

It is a condition that affects not just you and your quality of life but your family and friends and colleagues as well. How often have you had to miss a family party, not been able to make an important meeting, had to go to bed early or lost the first three days of your holiday just because of your migraine?

By its very nature, migraine is unpredictable. We all like to feel in control of our lives but migraine can strike at any time and often at the most inopportune time. The more you, as an individual, understand about your migraine and how it affects you, the greater chance you have of being able to control your migraine. Or at least feel in control of it some of the time if not all of the time.

DEFINING MIGRAINE

*I think that the headaches I get might be migraines but I'm
not really sure what the symptoms of a migraine are.
What actually is a migraine?*

Migraine is *not* 'just a headache'; it is a neurological condition
that research has shown is associated with a series of complex
changes that occur within the brain and brainstem. These changes
are a bit like a biochemical waterfall that, once started, is difficult to
stop and they generate all the symptoms that make a migraine (see
Figure 2.1).

It is an episodic condition – that is to say, it can occur now and
again. This frequency may be once a week, once a month or even once
a year. The frequency will vary from time to time as well as from person to person.

Migraine may occur with or without aura. About 10% of people
who get migraine get an aura. The most common aura is visual but
other aura symptoms include pins and needles and tingling or
numbness.

An attack stops you doing the things you want to do. It does this
because moving about will make the headache worse. Migraine might
make you feel sick (nauseated) or actually vomit. Light and sound
often make the headache feel worse. You just want to keep still until
the attack has gone.

*My GP says I have an aura with my migraine. What does
he mean?*

An aura is a collection of neurological symptoms that occur before
the start of the headache or as the headache starts. The aura is
usually followed by a 'high-impact' headache, less often with a 'low-
impact' headache or no headache at all. The aura affects up to 10% of
people with migraine, and can vary from person to person and from
attack to attack. Auras can be: visual (3.3%) – for example, flashing

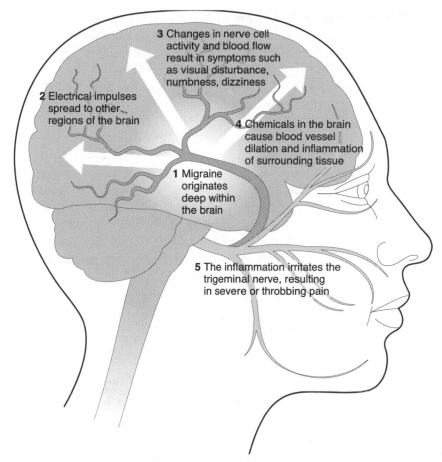

Figure 2.1 Migraine and the brain: the series of steps that are thought to lead to all the symptoms of a migraine attack.
(Adapted from *Target Migraine*, 2000, published by ABPI, London)

lights or blind spots; sensorimotor (1.2%) – for example, a sensation of numbness or tingling; or both (1.3%). It generally lasts between 5 and 60 minutes and settles completely at the end of that time.

My friend gets flashing lights when she gets migraine, but when my migraine starts I lose half of each word on the page. Are they both an aura?

Yes, they are. A visual aura is often described as flashing lights or zigzag lines that may appear as a small dot that grows and

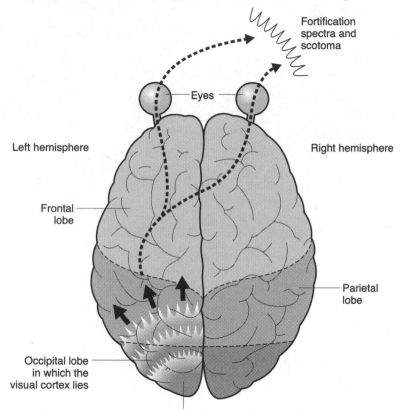

Figure 2.2 A view of the surface of the brain, showing the waves of change that have been identified and are thought to be responsible for the range of symptoms experienced during a migraine attack.
(Adapted from *Target Migraine*, 2000, published by APBI, London)

expands as the aura develops and evolves. It then slowly settles and disappears as vision returns to normal. Figure 2.2 shows the brain in relation to these visual effects.

Other people describe a distortion of the vision, such as half an object slipping, like a Picasso picture. Other people say that they can see only part of whatever it is that they are looking at.

Sometimes I just get flashing lights but at other times I get odd sensations or feelings at the same time that my vision goes funny. Should I be worried about this?

The aura can vary from attack to attack, but in general the overall pattern tends to be similar. It is possible to have symptoms that can be 'sensory', meaning that there is an alteration in sensation or feeling. This can be pins and needles or a tingling, which are called 'positive symptoms', or numbness, which is a 'negative symptom'.

It can affect any part of the body and is usually one-sided, affecting either side. It can start anywhere but often begins with the fingers or toes and spreads slowly upwards.

My aura usually lasts about 20 minutes but my sister says hers lasts an hour. Why are we different?

As you and your sister have found, the aura can last for a few minutes up to 60 minutes. The symptoms tend to develop over time and then settle completely. In most instances it leads straight into the headache phase of the attack. In some people, though, there can be a gap of up to an hour before the headache starts.

My mother always used to get a headache after her aura but since she went through 'the change' she still gets the flashing lights but rarely gets a headache. Why is that?

This can happen with some people as they get older. It is not always easy to predict whether it will happen to you. It is called *aura without headache*, and tends to occur in women at or around the time of the menopause. As your mother has found, there might be a very mild headache or no headache at all.

The specialist said to me that I have a migrainous headache, not IHS migraine. What does he mean?

'IHS' stands for the International Headache Society. A group of experts, in 1988, formed a committee that created a classification system that defines the different types of headaches. In this way, no matter where in the world a headache specialist or researcher is, the terminology is the same; results can be compared easily and used to further knowledge and develop better treatments.

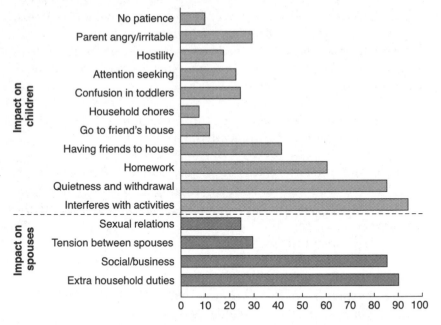

Figure 2.3 How attacks can affect you the migraine sufferer and your family relationships.
(Adapted from *Target Migraine*, 2000, published by ABPI, London)

The classification was revised in 2004 and acts as a guide to diagnosis for all patients who experience headache and their associated symptoms. There are dozens, if not hundreds, of different types of headache.

Headache tends to be a spectrum, the boundaries between different headache types tending to blur. Using the phrase 'migrainous headache' suggests that you have some but not all of the features of migraine to fulfil the IHS criteria. This potentially has implications for thinking about treatment options and evaluating your response to particular treatments tried.

What are the IHS criteria for diagnosing migraine?

The International Headache Society is quite clear and specific about what it takes to diagnose migraine. The criteria include a headache that is one-sided, moderate to severe in intensity, throbbing in quality and made worse by normal day-to-day activity. It is associated with nausea and/or vomiting and sensitivity to light and sound. It is episodic (occurs from time to time) and lasts from 4 to 72 hours.

The IHS suggests that, to fulfil the criteria for diagnosis, at least two of the following symptoms have to be present:

- unilateral (one-sided)
- pulsating
- moderate or severe in intensity
- aggravated by or causing avoidance of routine physical activity

and at least one of the following symptoms:

- nausea and/or vomiting
- sensitivity to light and sound (photophobia and phonophobia)

In the real world, you may have any combination of these symptoms but not necessarily all of them all of the time. In general terms, a 'high-impact' headache (one that has considerable effect on you) tends to be a migraine headache because it stops you doing the things that you want to do and need to do. Figure 2.3 shows how wide-ranging the impact of migraine is – it affects not just you but all the people around you.

TYPES OF MIGRAINE

I hadn't realised that there was more than one type of migraine. What are the main types?

There are lots of different types of migraine, the most common being *migraine without aura* (MOA). About 10% of migraine sufferers have *migraine with aura* (MA). There are even times when the aura can occur without the headache.

Then there are *basilar-type migraine, retinal migraine* and *familial hemiplegic migraine*. You could even have *menstrual migraine* (MM) or *menstrually associated migraine* (MAM); these two types are discussed in Chapter 15.

How are common and classical migraine different?

Common migraine, which is the type that affects most migraine sufferers, is now called *migraine without aura*. It is what it says it is: a migraine attack without aura symptoms.

Migraine is a condition that has an impact on your quality of life (QOL). The headache of migraine is a high-impact headache – one that stops you doing the things that you want to do or need to do. It is associated with nausea and/or vomiting, sensitivity to light and sound and possibly to smell, and with the need to keep still in the presence of these symptoms.

Classical migraine is now called *migraine with aura*. This affects about 1 in 10 migraine sufferers.

Aura is usually a visual disturbance, but may be associated with disturbance of sensation as well as other possible symptoms that usually occur before the headache and settle completely after 5 to 60 minutes.

The terms 'common' and 'classical' have fallen out of favour since the International Headache Society (IHS) developed a formal classification of headache disorders in 1988. Some doctors still use the terms 'common' and 'classical' but headache specialists refer to migraine by using the newer phrases of migraine with and without aura.

Why is it better to avoid the phrase 'classical' when referring to migraine?

This is to reduce confusion as to what is meant by the term 'classical'. Does it mean 'straight out of the textbook' or is it 'a migraine attack occurring with an aura'? Using the phrase 'migraine with aura' is absolutely clear and avoids any potential confusion.

I don't think I get migraine because I never get any flashing lights. Am I right?

If you do not get flashing lights, all it means is that you do not get an aura. Only 10% of migraine sufferers actually get an aura, so you don't have to experience this to have migraine. Migraine is a high-impact headache that makes you feel unwell and stops you doing what you want, or need, to do.

My friend's daughter seems to have migraines at different times, with no obvious cause or trigger. What brings on a migraine attack?

Answering that question is difficult. The answer varies depending on whether we take the pragmatic holistic approach or the scientific perspective.

Everyone is different and will say that X or Y causes their migraine, but not every time. The X and Y seem to be different for different people, at different times and in different circumstances. Some things cause problems for some of the people some of the time but not all of the people all of the time.

For more information on the migraine threshold and diet and lifestyle issues, see Chapter 7.

I can't figure out why I get a migraine some times and not at others. How can I find out what brings on my migraine?

You need to understand about your own migraine threshold – the point at which a migraine attack is more likely to occur – and what triggers affect your threshold. It helps to know how each trigger will tend to push your threshold down and nudge it closer to the point at which a migraine attack will inevitably occur. In any one person the combination of triggers that inevitably lead to a migraine will vary from day to day and month to month.

Despite this, there are some triggers that affect people every time they are exposed to it. Very bright sunlight flickering through trees on the roadside will always trigger a migraine in some people or eating citrus fruits or particular smells in others. That's the trouble with 'rules' – they are there to be broken!

Most of you will already know the things that always cause a migraine for you. I am not keen on suggesting that people keep detailed diaries, as this tends to focus too much on negative detail rather than taking positive steps. (For more ideas and suggestions on self-help, see Chapter 7.)

The headaches I get aren't always quite the same but they are pretty nasty. Are all my headaches migraines?

There are many different types of headaches and you can experience different headaches at different times. Migraine is a high-impact headache that may or may not be associated with aura.

Some people get just one sort of headache whereas others may experience several different headaches at different times. Working out exactly what headaches you get can be difficult and may take time, or several visits to your GP or a specialist.

Deciding which sort of headache you have is about understanding where you get your headache, what sort of head pain you experience and what sort of symptoms you get with your headache. Other important features include how long the headache lasts as well as how often you get your headache.

Next time you get your headache, write down what happens and how you feel. As with many unpleasant experiences, all you want to do is forget it as quickly as possible, so the best time to record what happens is while you are getting your headache or immediately after it has gone.

Often my migraines last for only a few hours but they can also last for more than a day. How long does a typical migraine last?

A typical migraine – that is, an IHS migraine – lasts from 4 to 72 hours in adults. This may vary from person to person and from attack to attack. The attack has a series of phases or stages. You may experience some of these phases some of the time, or all of the phases all of the time. The premonitory, or warning, phase is the first part of the attack. This may or may not be followed by an aura that leads to the headache phase and is followed by the recovery phase. Figure 2.4 outlines the phases and how they affect you.

Sometimes part of my face goes numb during a migraine. Is this normal?

This sort of symptom can occur during the aura or the headache phase of the migraine attack. It is part of the migraine, and does not cause any concern provided it settles before the headache does. If it extends beyond the headache phase, an assessment by a specialist is probably a good idea, but often it is part and parcel of the migraine rather than due to any underlying non-migraine reason. (For information on potentially serious symptoms, see Chapter 5.)

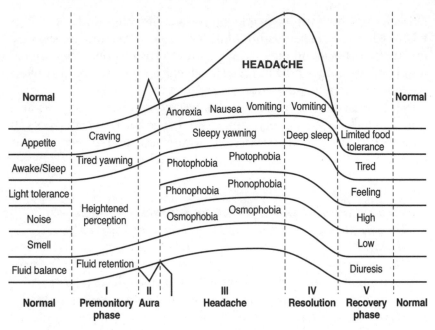

Figure 2.4 The phases of a migraine attack and the symptoms associated with each phase .
(Adapted from J N Blau, 1992, 'Migraine: theories of pathogenesis',
Lancet vol. 339: 1202–7)

I've always had headaches from time to time but they seem to be getting worse. Should I be worried?

This is not an easy one to answer as it depends on what you mean by 'worse'. Do you mean the pain is more severe or that the headache is lasting longer or that you are getting more associated symptoms? Do you mean that the attacks are more frequent? Or do you mean that the treatment is not working as well?

The severity of the pain can and does vary from attack to attack and it is impossible to predict or anticipate how it will be. As you go from childhood to teens and then adulthood the pain will often become more significant and may last longer. The pattern of symptoms and the frequency that you get your headaches can evolve and change through your life, and may vary from time to time for good reasons and sometimes for no reason at all.

There are times when you get all the symptoms associated with migraine and other times when you get very few. Again, it is impossible to anticipate how and when and why. If you have any worries or concerns, do go and talk to your GP about them.

I'm a bit worried because my headaches seem to be happening more often and I don't know why. Can you reassure me?

The frequency of migraine attacks can vary for a wide range of reasons. A major factor is where your migraine threshold is: the higher the threshold, the less likely you are to get a migraine. The more potential triggers you expose yourself to, the lower your threshold and the more likely you are to get a migraine. Stress is often the thing that does the most to push your threshold down, but other factors can be just as important.

If you feel that you are exposing yourself to a variety of triggers, there is probably no need for concern; just think about what you can do to raise your migraine threshold. If you feel there are few or no triggers in your life at the moment, and you are not getting any new or different symptoms with your migraine, it is unlikely that you should be concerned, but you might want to see your GP about what you can do to reduce the frequency of your attacks.

If, however, you are experiencing new or different symptoms, it is probably wise to go and talk to your GP about them and make sure there is nothing to worry about. It may be that all you need is to think about preventative treatment, which your GP can discuss with you.

For more information about preventative treatment options, see Chapter 12.

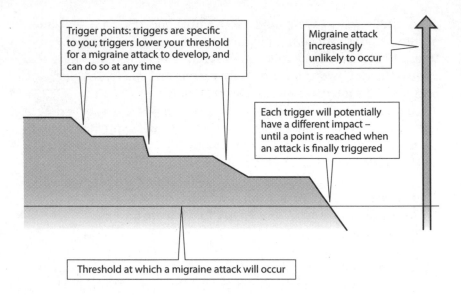

Figure 2.5 How triggers can come together to push down your migraine threshold to the point where an attack is likely to result.

What is the typical number of migraines that most people have in a month or a year?

There is no 'right' answer to that question. The frequency can vary from time to time and from person to person. Some people can get a migraine a week, others a migraine a month and others may get only one or two a year. And some people can go for a few weeks with no attacks, followed by a week or so with several attacks.

The length of an attack can vary, the attack being as short as a few hours or as long as three days. It is sometimes more helpful to think about *migraine days* rather than the number of attacks. This measure is useful in trying to assess the response to both acute treatment and preventative treatment. The goal in assessing a response to treatment is to reduce the total number of headache days.

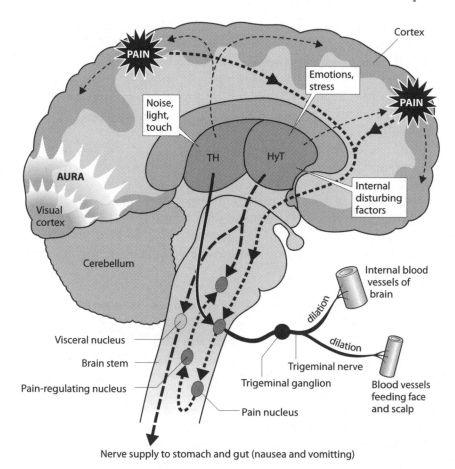

Figure 2.6 A vertical section of the brain, showing the structures in the brain and how they interact with each other during a migraine attack. TH is the thalamus, which is involved in noise, light and touch; HyT is the hypothalamus, which is involved in emotion and stress and in controlling internal factors and processes.
(Adapted from J N Blau, 1992, 'Migraine: theories of pathogenesis', *Lancet* vol. 339: 1202–7)

I've never had two migraines 'set off' by the same trigger in the same week. Does this mean that I'm briefly immune to the trigger by having the first attack?

The simple answer is 'No'. Your migraine has occurred because your threshold dropped to the point at which a migraine became inevitable.

Different factors or 'triggers' come together, usually in a random fashion, and push the threshold down. These factors often have different effects at different times, depending on where your threshold is and in which mix the triggers come together. This is probably why you feel that different triggers are responsible. Figure 2.5 outlines how this can happen.

For more information on the migraine threshold and self-help, see Chapter 7.

What is happening to me when I get a migraine attack?

Not an easy question to answer! Science is making small steps in understanding more about what is going on within the brain during a migraine attack. There are complex changes to chemicals (neurotransmitters) within the brain that affect the brain and the blood vessels in the brain as well as the whole nervous system. These changes then lead to the symptoms that you experience during a migraine attack. Figure 2.6 outlines the pathways in the brain.

I have been reading about chemicals in the brain and migraine. What is serotonin?

Serotonin is one of several neurotransmitters involved in the migraine attack. It is also referred to as 5-HT. There are two 5-HT receptor subtypes located in blood vessels in the brain: 5-HT_{1B} and 5-HT_{1D}. Activating these receptors causes a constriction of the blood vessel.

Figure 2.7 shows how these 5-HT receptors link together and lead to the changes in migraine.

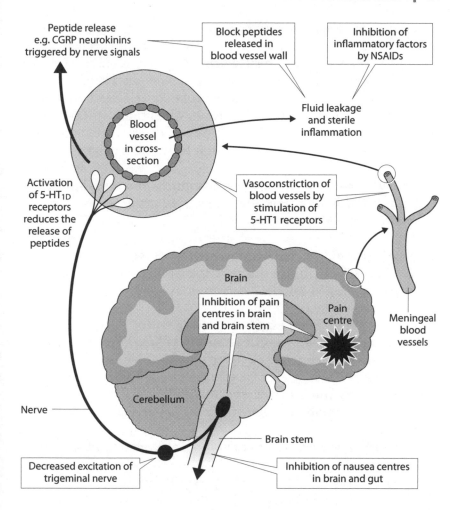

Figure 2.7 A vertical section of the brain, showing the location of serotonin (5-HT) receptors and how they link together in migraine.
(Adapted from *Target Migraine*, 2000, published by ABPI, London)

What is CGRP and what does it do?

CGRP – calcitonin gene-related peptide – is a molecule that causes dilatation (widening) of blood vessels in the brain and also releases other chemicals (such as neurokinins) that lead to 'sterile' inflammation in the membrane around the brain. Any drug that mimics serotonin will block their release and hence prevent the vessel from dilating, or constrict the vessel if it has already dilated.

I thought that migraines occurred mainly in women but I've discovered that men have them, too. Is migraine more common in men or women?

Migraine is more common in women, by about 3 to 1. This difference seems to develop during and after puberty; until then boys and girls are affected equally.

Both my partner and I suffer from migraines. Does this mean that our children will be more likely to have them, too?

Yes, they are more likely to develop migraines than if neither you nor your partner suffered from them.
For more information on heredity, see Chapter 6.

How do I know whether I'm having an ordinary headache or a migraine?

With an ordinary headache you will usually be able to carry on with what you are doing. Migraine will make you want to keep still and, as it gets worse, you may want to lie down or retreat to a dark, quiet room.

I've decided to see my GP about my headaches. How will she decide whether they are migraines or something else more serious?

Your GP will ask you a variety of questions about your headache and any symptoms associated with it. Deciding what sort of headache you have is about pattern recognition. If your headache fits into a specific pattern, that is the probable diagnosis. Making sure your headache is not serious or sinister means ruling out symptoms that cause concern.

If you want more information about the sorts of questions that your GP or specialist might ask you, see Chapter 10.

My GP said that my migraines are just that – that there are no 'red flags'. What does he mean by 'red flags'?

'Red flags' are the symptoms that may suggest a more serious cause for the headache. Sometimes these red flags have to be viewed in the context of your previous symptoms and sometimes they are important irrespective of your previous symptoms.

For more information on 'red flags', see Chapter 5.

Sometimes I can go several weeks without a migraine and then I have two or three in a week. Why is this?

How often you get migraine can and does vary. Migraine is, by its nature, unpredictable, and occurs now and again. 'Now and again' may be once a week, once a month or several times a year. If your threshold is low for any reason, it does not take much to keep pushing you over the edge into a migraine.

When you say two or three in a week, do you mean separate headache days or are you getting a headache for two to three consecutive days? The latter means your attack is lasting longer rather than occurring more frequently.

The pain is always worse on the right side of my forehead. Why is this?

In migraine the pain is often, but not always, one-sided. Even if the pain starts on one side, though, it can move to the other side during an attack, or from attack to attack. If the pain affects both sides, the pain will often be worse on one side than the other. Different people have different experiences with where they get their headache – your headache just happens to be right-sided.

My mother's migraines seem to have got better lately. Will my migraines get better as I get older?

In most people, migraines tend to get better as you get older. The pain may get less severe, the associated symptoms may get less intense, and the attacks may occur less often or stop completely.

In some women, attacks become more frequent around the time of the menopause. In others they occur less often and stop altogether.

So it is not unreasonable to expect your migraines to get better as you get older but, unfortunately, it is by no means guaranteed.

Even after the pain has gone, it still takes me another day or so to feel better. I feel absolutely washed out, tired and listless. Is this normal?

What you describe is commonly called the *recovery phase*, which is the final part of the migraine attack. This is the time when the brain is completing its recovery from the attack and the brain is slowly returning to normal function.

The symptoms people experience during this phase vary from person to person and sometimes from attack to attack. The length of time that the symptoms last can also vary.

My cousin says that her doctor told her that she probably has basilar migraine. What on earth is that?

Basilar migraine is now referred to as *basilar-type migraine*. This is a type of migraine that is associated with a very specific set of aura symptoms. These aura symptoms can be quite dramatic and as a result quite frightening, especially when they occur for the first time. The headache that follows fulfils the criteria for the IHS classification of migraine without aura (described earlier in this chapter).

The aura has to include at least two of the following symptoms:

- dysarthria – the speech is slurred, and there is a difficulty saying words

- vertigo – a sensation of spinning or turning

- tinnitus – a ringing or buzzing in the ears

- phonophobia – sensitivity to sound (also referred to as hyperacusia)

- diplopia – double vision

- visual symptoms occurring at both sides of your visual field, either close to the nose or close to the temple

- ataxia – an unsteadiness or clumsiness when moving your arms or legs

- decreased level of consciousness

- paraesthesiae – abnormal skin sensations that include tingling and numbness that are felt on both sides at the same time

These symptoms may develop individually, in isolation, or in sequence over 5 to 60 minutes, and resolve completely before the headache starts.

My son tells me that he has retinal migraine. Can you explain what that is?

Retinal migraine is a form of migraine in which the visual disturbance of the aura affects only one eye. The visual auras are 'positive' with flashing or zigzag lights and lines or spots, or 'negative' with blind spots (scotomata) or a blindness affecting part of the field of vision in one eye such as a hemianopia or quadrantonopia (half or a quarter of the field of vision). The headache that follows fulfils the IHS criteria for migraine without aura (discussed earlier in this chapter).

I have been told that I have retinal migraine. How do I know something more serious is not causing my symptoms?

By 'serious' do you mean something wrong in the brain? Ruling out a possibly serious cause in this situation is based on assessing the symptoms you experience and combining that with an adequate examination of your eyes and a neurological assessment. That assessment may or may not include a brain scan, which would be able to identify a specific 'structural', or organic, cause for your symptoms.

When symptoms affect one side and particularly if they always affect the same side, a structural cause may need to be excluded before the benign nature of the symptom can be accepted. Benign 'primary' headaches are much more likely than a more serious 'secondary' headache.

For more information on 'red flags' regarding possibly serious causes of headache, see Chapter 5.

I have had episodes in which I was unable to move my arm, at the same time as I had my normal migraine aura. What sort of migraine is this?

An inability to physically move your arm suggests a true paralysis, or *paresis*, which is different from a feeling of heaviness. This 'motor weakness' is suggestive of a form of migraine known as *hemiplegic migraine*, which indicates paralysis down one side. If you have relatives who experience this form of migraine, it is called *familial hemiplegic migraine*; if not, it is referred to as *sporadic hemiplegic migraine*.

The paralysis has to be accompanied by at least one of the following:

- fully reversible visual symptoms

- fully reversible sensory symptoms (see the fourth answer in this chapter)

- fully reversible speech disturbance

and at least two of the following:

- at least one aura symptom develops over about 5 minutes and/or different symptoms occur in succession

- each aura symptom lasts more than about 5 minutes but less than 24 hours

- headache fulfilling the IHS criteria for migraine without aura (see earlier in this chapter), beginning during the aura or within 60 minutes of the aura starting

My cousin has been told she has familial hemiplegic migraine. Could I develop the same sort of migraine?

It is possible, if you have a first- or second-degree relative (parent, sibling, aunt, uncle, cousin) who has migraine with aura with 'motor weakness'. Familial hemiplegic migraine has been linked to a specific chromosome abnormality.

For more information on chromosomes and migraine, look in Chapter 6.

There are times when my arm feels heavy but I can move it. Is this a type of paralysis?

No, it isn't. Paralysis means being completely unable to move a part of your body, rather than a sensation of not wanting to or of it feeling heavy.

Can migraine last for longer than 72 hours?

Yes, it can but, fortunately, not often. It may be as a result of the overuse of medication or the prolongation of an attack to four days from three days when using triptans that allow recurrence of headache symptoms. Medication overuse headache is discussed in Chapter 3 and triptans are discussed in Chapter 11.

Is it possible to get a stroke as a result of migraine?

Yes, it is possible to have a stroke as a result of migraine; it is confirmed on brain imaging, usually a CT scan. Some studies have found that women under the age of 45 who have migraine have an increased risk of stroke. The risk is greater in women who have aura.

The important thing to remember is that the absolute risk, or the chance of a stroke occurring, is very, very low indeed. Current figures suggest that 1 to 3 per 100,000 women under the age of 35 years may have an ischaemic stroke. This increases slightly to 10 per 100,000 women over the age of 35. A three-fold increase in this risk is still very few people.

If you have any concerns about the risk of stroke, think first about exercising regularly, eating a healthy diet, not smoking and having your blood pressure checked, and perhaps consider what your weight is. If you need any more advice, have a chat with your practice nurse or GP. (For more information about women's health, see Chapters 7 and 15.)

3 | Headaches that are not migraine

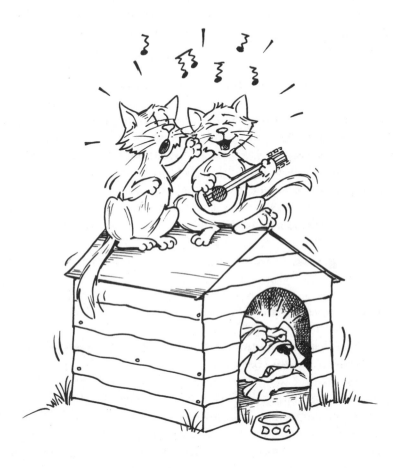

Headaches are not always easy to label. The same person may experience more than one type of headache. One type of headache may develop and evolve over time to a different sort of headache. So it can be quite challenging for any doctor – expert or not – to decide exactly what your headache is at the initial consultation or assessment.

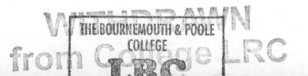

Different headaches are identified and separated by the nature, description, site and severity of the pain as well as the wide range of symptoms associated with the pain. In crude terms, it is about pattern recognition – but there are exceptions to every rule and not all the patterns fit neatly in to the available 'diagnostic boxes'.

This chapter discusses tension-type headache, chronic daily headache, medication overuse headache and cluster headache. Some of the more idiosyncratic and less common headaches are discussed in Chapter 4.

Before going to see your GP or headache specialist about your headache symptoms, spend some time writing down exactly where you get your headache, what it feels like and what symptoms you get with it. Think about what might bring on your headache or ease the symptoms you experience. If you have thought about these things in advance, it should make it easier to answer the questions you will be asked. This is discussed further in Chapter 9, and aspects of your headaches to consider are listed in Chapter 10.

For information on recognising 'red flag' symptoms, see Chapter 5.

TENSION-TYPE HEADACHE

I have looked on the internet and I think I have a tension headache. How can I be sure?

Tension-type headache (TTH) tends to be described as tightness, or a band-like pressure. It is not usually associated with any of the migraine symptoms, such as nausea, vomiting or sensitivity to light or sound. Moreover, you can usually carry on with your daily activities and will usually respond to a *single* dose of a simple painkiller, provided it is used only occasionally. Tension-type headache tends to last for several hours over several days, for days or weeks, and may even come on at the same sort of time in the day.

***My headache is just like a tight band round my head.
What sort of headache could it be?***

A band-like headache is usually thought to be a tension-type headache (TTH). This can only really be confirmed by checking what, if any, other symptoms you experience with your headache. Tension-type headache tends to be diagnosed by what is missing as much as by what is present in terms of symptoms. If you do not have any symptoms of nausea or sensitivity to light, it is more likely that you have TTH rather than migraine.

***My headache gets worse through the day, but I never have
to go to bed with them like my sister does. What sort of
headache do I have?***

A ttaching a label with only this much information is not really possible. In general terms, though, if you can carry on doing what you want or need to do, it is more likely that it is a low-impact headache such as a tension-type headache. The fact that it gets worse through the day also suggests that this may be a tension-type headache.

If you answer 'No' to the following questions, it is more likely to be tension-type headache:

- Do you ever feel sick with this headache?

- Do you ever need to keep still with your headache or lie down?

- Do you ever feel as though you need to wear tinted glasses with your headache or avoid bright lights?

- Is the pain only ever on one side?

- Is it a throbbing, pounding headache?

If you can say 'Yes' to one or more of the questions, you have some migrainous features to your headache. The more you can say 'Yes', the more likely that the headache is migraine.

> *Sometimes I feel a bit sick with my headache but don't usually have to go to bed. About once a month, though, I feel really sick with the headache and have to go to bed with it. Do I have one headache or two different headaches?*

You may well have two different types of headache, and I sometimes refer to this as a mixed-picture headache. The high-impact headache that you get once a month is probably migraine. If your high-impact headache *is* migraine, it is possible that you will feel nauseated or a bit light-sensitive with a low-impact headache. Your other headache, which is a low-impact headache, and doesn't send you to bed, is probably a tension-type headache.

> *On some days I get my normal headache and other times I get a headache that is so bad I have to go to bed. Are these different headaches?*

They may be two completely different but separate headaches or be slightly different headaches that may be linked. If you read on, you may be able to work out what sort of headache you have.

If you get an occasional headache that lasts a few hours every now and again and is of low impact, this is probably a tension-type headache. If you get a headache that lasts a few hours most days, we need to think about it a bit more. It could be a chronic tension-type headache, a chronic daily headache or even a medication overuse headache.

A 'go to bed' headache that happens every now and again is usually migraine. A 'go to bed' headache that happens regularly with a less severe headache in between needs a little more thought and assessment.

If you are taking some sort of painkiller most days, it is possible that you have medication overuse headache. This can happen if too many painkillers are taken to treat headache symptoms.

How to deal with these different types of headache is discussed in Chapters 11, 12 and 13.

What I want to know is why, on a bright day, I can wear tinted glasses but on a really sunny day I have to wear very dark glasses or I get a migraine?

If you get regular or frequent migraine, it is not unusual to be a little light-sensitive in between attacks. Some people are more sensitive than others, some people are light-sensitive all of the time and some just in the few hours or days leading up to their next attack. It is this light sensitivity that may cause the headache to get worse or drop your migraine threshold to the point that a migraine is triggered.

You need to use the tinted glasses between attacks as a result of this light sensitivity that gets magnified during the attack, so you then move on to dark glasses.

CHRONIC DAILY HEADACHE AND MEDICATION OVERUSE HEADACHE

My son's GP says that he has chronic daily headache. What is that?

'Chronic daily headache' (CDH) is a label applied to a collection of different types of headache rather than a diagnosis in the way that migraine or cluster headache are. It describes a headache that occurs on more days than it is absent. CDH usually happens on more than 15 days in each month, and is present for some part of most days. It is a descriptive phrase rather than a formal diagnosis.

I was involved in a car accident two years ago. I got a headache at the time but it seemed to settle after a few days. Then a week or two later it started again and I haven't had a headache-free day since. What is causing my headaches?

Making a diagnosis for someone with a daily headache is difficult without a lot more information:

- Did you get a bang to the head during the accident?

- Were you unconscious at any time?

- Did you suffer a neck injury or significant whiplash?

- Do you take any painkillers for your headache?

- If you do take painkillers, how often do you take them?

Any bang to the head can lead to a headache that is defined as a post-traumatic headache. It is not serious or 'sinister' and usually settles six to eight weeks after the injury but can persist for as long as two years. A headache that develops rapidly in the first few hours or days after a head injury is much more likely to give cause for concern than one that has persisted for months or years. See Chapter 5 for information on serious or sinister causes of headache.

The other issue is about your use of medication, which may have switched an episodic (occasional) post-traumatic headache to a medication overuse headache (MOH). If this seems to be the case, you should talk to your GP about ways to solve the problem (see Chapter 13 for information on tackling MOH).

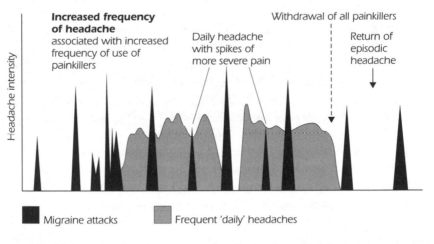

Figure 3.1 Medication overuse headache: how the changing use of painkillers can affect headache frequency.

*A colleague suffers a lot – virtually every day – with what
seems to be a migraine. Is it possible to get a migraine
every day?*

No, migraine is by definition an episodic headache – it happens
from time to time. Migraine cannot and does not occur every day
for days and days or weeks and weeks. Your colleague may have
migraine as part of a *mixed picture headache*, with some headache-free
days, or she may have chronic daily headache (CDH) or medication
overuse headache (MOH) with 'breakthrough' migrainous symptoms
(see Figure 3.1).

*What is the difference between a chronic daily headache
and a medication overuse headache?*

Chronic daily headache (CDH) is a collective term loosely applied
to a variety of headache types – and medication overuse
headache (MOH) is one of them. The diagnosis of MOH can be
confirmed only when all the acute headache treatments (painkillers
and/or triptans) are stopped completely for at least six to eight weeks
and the headache improves to a significant degree.

For advice on how to try to change a medication overuse headache
back to an episodic headache, have look at Chapter 13.

*I use ibuprofen to get rid of my headache. I only take a
couple every day, but I was looking on the internet last week
and it said taking painkillers every day might make my
headache worse. Can that really be right?*

Yes, that is right. It is not advisable to take painkillers every day to
treat headache symptoms. Any painkiller taken on a daily or
near-daily basis may, in a susceptible individual, lead to daily
headache rather than stop your headaches. This is more likely to happen if you take one or two tablets every day than four doses in one day
once in the week.

Table 3.1 Over-the-counter preparations containing codeine

Name of preparation	Codeine content
Boots Tension Headache Relief	10 mg
Nurofen Plus	12.8 mg
Panadol Ultra	12.8 mg
Paracodol	8 mg
Phensic Dual Action	8 mg
Propain	10 mg
Solpadeine Plus	8 mg
Solpaflex	12.8 mg
Syndol	10 mg
Veganin	6.8 mg

My doctor said that, provided I avoid painkillers with codeine in them, I can't get a drug-related headache. Is that right?

Yes and no. Painkillers containing codeine will lead more easily to a medication overuse headache but any painkiller taken regularly over time has the potential to do this. There is codeine in many preparations that you can buy over the counter (without a prescription), so remember to read the labels, just to be sure. Table 3.1 lists some of the common over-the-counter preparations that contain codeine.

I get a headache every day and am finding it difficult to put up with. Why does this happen?

A daily headache can be caused by many things. It might be what is called a 'primary headache' such as tension-type headache, chronic daily headache or cluster headache. It might be a 'secondary headache' resulting from another disease process, such as diabetes or an overactive thyroid, for example.

You need to visit your doctor to see if they can identify your headache. The GP or a specialist will ask you a series of questions to assess your symptoms and decide what, if any, investigations are needed. Deciding what sort of headache you have is about weighing up the range of symptoms in combination with the results of any examination or investigations. A diagnosis is sometimes made on the basis of your history alone and confirmed by the results of normal tests.

Once the doctor knows what type of headache you have, the right steps can be taken to treat it. For more information on managing headaches, see Chapters 11, 12 and 13.

I am getting a migraine every day but nothing I take for it seems to work any more. Why is this?

First of all, migraine cannot and does not occur every day, for days and days and days. Migraine is an episodic headache that occurs every now and again. Some of your daily headaches might be migraine but not all of them.

If you use painkillers to treat all your headaches and take those painkillers on most days, it is possible that your headache is a medication overuse headache (MOH). MOH develops as your treatment becomes less and less effective against your headache and you try stronger and stronger painkillers to no avail. Your headache happens more and more often, so you take more and more painkillers. (See Figure 3.1.)

You need to talk to your doctor about the problem so that, between you, you can find a way to solve the problem. For advice on how to change your MOH back to an episodic headache, see Chapter 13.

I get this pressure headache every day. It doesn't last all day but it has been there for some of the day for the last three months. Why will it just not go away?

A pressure headache in the absence of more typical migraine symptoms is probably a tension-type headache (TTH). Having a daily headache suggests a chronic TTH – provided you are not overusing painkillers. If you *are* overusing painkillers, you have a medication overuse headache and your headache will not improve until you stop taking them. (How you can do this is discussed in Chapter 13.)

If you aren't using painkillers regularly, you may need to think about diet and lifestyle changes to raise your headache threshold or consider a preventative drug to try to settle the headache symptoms. Talk to your GP about the options that are available.

See Chapters 11 and 12, which look at how to treat different types of headaches, or Chapter 7, to find ways of raising your headache threshold.

My specialist told me I have a medication overuse headache. He said that it has happened because I take too many painkillers. I don't take more than the recommended dose, so how can that be?

There are lots of theories about how this might happen. In general terms, the pain receptors within the brain change in some way and, as a result of that change, they become oversensitive, and instead of being 'switched off' by the painkiller are in some way kept 'switched on'.

Any painkiller can cause this shift in receptor response. What seems to be important is how often you are taking the painkillers to treat headache symptoms. Research evidence suggests that it is how many days in the week that you take the tablets, rather than how many tablets you take in the day, that leads to the shift in pain receptor response. The more regularly you take them, the more likely they are to lead to a medication overuse headache.

My doctor told me I have a medication overuse headache. I don't think I use too much medication, so how did it happen?

Medication overuse headache (MOH) tends to creep up on you. You start off getting headaches every now and again. Some of them are worse than others. You try different tablets but nothing seems to work. You get something a bit stronger from the pharmacy; or you might go to your GP who suggests a stronger painkiller and says, 'It's fine provided you don't exceed the maximum dose' – and sometimes the headache goes away and sometimes it doesn't.

Before you know it, you seem to have a dull nagging headache every day (see Figure 3.1). It's not really very bad but you get used to it being there. You almost learn to live with it but then you start to get some really bad headaches for a day or perhaps two. You think about going back to the doctor but they settle down, life is too busy and you just reach for the pills.

Anyone who takes regular painkillers to treat headache symptoms runs the risk of eventually feeding the headache rather than relieving it. Not everybody is affected in this way, and it is impossible to predict who might be affected. It can happen all too easily in some of the people some of the time.

Look at Chapter 7 for suggestions on how to raise your headache threshold or Chapter 12 for drugs that might reduce the number of headache days you have. Your GP or practice nurse should be able to offer you some help or support while you try to make changes. Tackling MOH is dealt with in Chapter 13.

My GP has told me that I should stop taking so many painkillers. I just can't imagine surviving without them. What should I do?

It is not uncommon to feel 'I just can't do without my tablets' or 'I don't take too many because I never take more than it says on the pack'. But if you are taking tablets on a daily or near-daily basis, you may be feeding the headache rather than relieving it.

The only way to find out if this is the case is to stop all the painkillers for at least six to eight weeks, often longer. If medication overuse is the cause of your headache, you should eventually experience a significant improvement in your headache symptoms or they may even settle completely. To begin with, though, you will probably need to talk to your GP about ways to cope without painkillers. This is discussed in more detail in Chapter 13; see also Chapter 12 if you want to take a preventative drug to help reduce the number of headache days.

> **My GP says I must not take too many painkillers, but if my headache is happening every day how can I get rid of it without taking them?**

How often were you getting your headache three months ago, or six months ago, or perhaps a year ago? If your answer is 'A lot less often than now', you need to think about how your use of painkillers has changed. If they have slowly but definitely increased, it is quite likely that the painkillers are *causing* the problem now rather than solving it.

The only way to get rid of the headache in the short to medium term is to stop all the painkillers. You cannot take any painkillers no matter how bad the headache gets during this 'washout' phase of treatment. Talk to your GP about what other drugs, that are not painkillers, you could use to treat the pain. (Look at Chapter 12 for advice on preventative drugs and Chapter 13 on tackling medication overuse headache.)

> **Syndol was the only drug that helped my headache but over the last few months it hasn't seemed to work so well, and I have to take them more often. What should I do?**

Drugs such as Syndol have several different active ingredients (Syndol has paracetamol, caffeine, codeine and doxylamine). When taken occasionally to treat headache, it can work quite well. If it stops working so well and you start taking it more regularly, over time it may lead to an increase in headaches.

As to what to do, you need to stop the painkillers for at least six to eight weeks. The headache may get worse before it gets better, but stopping the tablets is the only way to get back in control. Ask your GP what alternatives you can take in the meantime. (Look at Chapter

12 for advice on preventative drugs and Chapter 13 on tackling medication overuse headache.)

I seem to have a constant headache, and take several over-the-counter painkillers a day. How can I make the headaches stop?

If you are taking painkillers every day or even most days, it is possible that the painkillers are contributing to the headache. How often did you get your headaches when they first started? Did you take lots of different painkillers that seemed to work for a while and then they stopped working?

The only way to stop the headaches if they are caused by the painkillers is to stop the painkillers for a minimum of six to eight weeks. This means taking no headache medication, no matter how bad the headache gets during this 'washout' phase.

It may be that you need to see your GP for alternative pain treatment such as tricyclic antidepressants or anti-epileptic drugs. Both of these drugs are used to treat the pain in a variety of chronic (long-term) conditions without taking regular painkillers.

Look at Chapter 12 for more advice on preventative drugs and Chapter 13 on tackling MOH.

I have been to a neurologist and he has told me I should stop taking any painkillers or my headache will not get better. How can I do that?

The 'how' depends on what you feel you need to do to stop. We all lead busy, complex lives and have different worries, pressures and concerns, and we try to balance a host of demands on us.

Don't be afraid to ask for help from friends and family. It may be that you will need time off work, so go and see your GP or talk to your boss, or both! The only way to succeed is to plan carefully, choose the right time and take small steps so that you can stop for long enough to help the headaches get better.

*I have just seen my GP, who has told me my painkillers might
be causing my headaches. How will I manage if I stop them?*

If you can stop taking the painkillers, your medication overuse
headache will get better. It is one of those contradictions, as you
can confirm the diagnosis only if you stop the painkillers ... but you
don't want to stop the painkillers in case the headache does not get
better. If the diagnosis is right, you will get fewer headaches and the
ones that you do get will respond better to the treatment you use.

You and your GP need to think about other options during this
withdrawal or washout phase, that are not painkillers but will help
treat your symptoms. A variety of drugs are used to manage chronic
pain that will reduce the frequency and severity of your headache
symptoms. This might be a short-, medium- or long-term option.

For more information, see Chapters 12 and 13 on how to help
reduce the number of headache days.

*I have been told I have to stop my painkillers. I think I can do
that provided I have some time off work. What should I do?*

If you explain to your GP what you need to do, you should be able
to get a sick note to cover the time off you need. It is difficult to predict how long it will take but you should probably plan on two to three
weeks. It may be that you need a little less or a little more time.

*I am planning to stop taking painkillers for my headaches,
and the nurse told me that my headaches may get worse.
What can I do about this and might I get any other symptoms?*

Yes, the headache will often get worse before it gets better in this
situation but stopping the painkillers is the only way to make the
diagnosis.

The symptoms you get when stopping painkillers can vary dramatically from person to person. They may also vary depending on which
mix of painkillers you have been taking. You can probably expect to

feel sick and sometimes vomit. It is not unusual to experience mood swings and irritability. Some people have disturbed sleep as well.

Look at Chapter 12 for more advice on preventative drugs and Chapter 13 on tackling medication overuse headache. And you might be one of the lucky people who have no problems at all!

My GP gave me a triptan to treat my migraine. It used to work really well but now my headache seems to be lasting longer and seems to be coming back most days. Why is that?

Triptans can cause a medication overuse headache (MOH) in the same way that any other painkiller can. A triptan is just another headache treatment in that sense. Your headache may be a *triptan rebound headache*, and it will often recur at the same sort of time every day. You don't say exactly how often you get your headache: is it more or fewer than 15 days in each month?

If you are using more than eight to ten triptans a month, it is possible that, even if you don't have a triptan rebound headache now, if you carry on at this sort of dose level, you will have one in the not-too-distant future. The question to ask yourself is 'How many triptans am I taking each month?'; if the answer is more than 10 or 12, you probably have a triptan rebound headache.

For more advice on tackling MOH, have a look at Chapter 13.

My GP has said that I can't have more than six sumatriptan tablets on each prescription, but I use those up in 10 days. What can I do?

Your GP has a point in limiting your triptans to just six on each prescription as that way he can monitor how many you use. If you take too many, you run the risk of developing a triptan rebound headache or medication overuse headache (MOH).

If you used only six in a whole month, there would be less of a problem. But you say you are using six every 10 days, so you need to be thinking about whether you are using too many and seek further help. Talk to your GP about your difficulty and work out a way to minimise the number of tablets you have to take.

For more advice on treating your migraine, look at Chapter 11, or even Chapter 13 on tackling medication overuse headache.

> **How do I know if I am using too many triptans? I take one to get rid of the headache as soon as it starts. The headache gets better but comes back the next day, so I repeat the dose then. Is that too many?**

If you are getting one attack a month, you are not using too many. If, however, you are getting one attack every week, you might be using too many.

If you are using eight to ten triptans every month, you are at risk of the headaches getting more frequent as a result of the medication. If you are using 12 or more each month, it is even more likely that the tablets are contributing to the problem and you are developing a triptan rebound headache.

Talk to your doctor about how often the headaches come back and, together, you should be able to solve the problem.

CLUSTER HEADACHE AND OTHER TRIGEMINAL AUTONOMIC CEPHALALGIAS

Trigeminal autonomic cephalalgias (TACs) are a separate section within the International Headache Society classification and represent four different headache types:

- cluster headache, in an episodic or chronic form
- paroxysmal hemicrania in an episodic or chronic form
- short-lasting unilateral neuralgiform headache
- short-lasting unilateral neuralgiform headache attacks with conjunctival injection and tearing (SUNCT)

I'm not sure whether my headache is a migraine or a cluster type. How can I tell?

Migraine is a headache that stops you being able to do things. Migraine makes you want to keep still. Cluster headache, which can be as severe if not more severe than migraine, tends to stop you doing things but you will pace about because you cannot keep still. There is more about cluster headaches in the answers that follow.

I get this really bad pain several times a night. It is so bad I have to get up and pace about – I just can't keep still. What could it be?

It is possible that you are experiencing a bout of cluster headache. Cluster headache pain is very definitely one-sided and tends to make the sufferer agitated, unlike in migraine where the sufferer chooses to keep still.

Cluster headache is associated with other symptoms, including reddening and watering of the eye on the same side as the pain. The eye can become swollen and sometimes close a little. You may also get a runny nose on the same side as the pain or it may feel blocked.

Cluster headache lasts for 15 to 180 minutes whereas SUNCT lasts for only 5 to 240 seconds. Cluster headache will occur up to 8 times a day, whereas SUNCT occurs between 3 and 200 times a day.

I get a really bad headache that sits around my eye. Is this migraine or, as my GP suggested, cluster headache?

In order to answer this question I need more information:

- Is your headache always just around your eye, or does it spread further?

- Is your headache always just on one side, or does it spread to both sides?

- Does your eye go red and water on the same side as the headache?

- Is the pain a severe and intense stabbing pain, as opposed to a throbbing, pounding pain?

- Does your nose run or feel blocked on the same side as the pain?

A 'Yes' to some or all of these makes cluster headache more likely than migraine.

I also need to know how long the pain lasts and how often you get the pain each day. These two pieces of information will help determine exactly which headache you might have.

Every time I get this pain around my eye, it goes red and waters. It is really weird as my nose feels blocked as well. I could understand it if I was doing something that would make my eyes water, but it just comes out of the blue, and it is only on one side. What could it be? My GP is not sure and is sending me to see a specialist.

It sounds like cluster headache, but it could be any one of the four TACs listed above. They are not particularly common conditions and it is possible that your GP has not seen a patient with them before. Because it can be difficult to treat, sending you to a headache specialist is a good idea.

I get this pain that always affects my left eye, and sometimes it spreads to my forehead and temple. My eye waters and can close. I just want to bang my head when I get this pain it is so bad. What could be causing it?

Cluster headache is the most likely diagnosis, but I need to know how long the pain lasts to be absolutely sure. What causes it, though, is slightly more complex. During a cluster attack, changes occur in a very specific part of the brain called the posterior hypothal-amic grey matter. There is no doubt that this is part of the process of cluster headache but what actually triggers, or sets off, each attack is still not absolutely certain.

For information on how to treat cluster headache, see Chapters 11 and 12, or have a look at the OUCH UK website (details in Appendix 1).

I get cluster headache that lasts for a few weeks at a time. Could it last longer than it does now?

The simple answer to that is 'Yes, possibly'. *Episodic cluster headache* usually occurs for several weeks, often up to three months at a time. The International Headache Society (IHS) classification states that cluster periods last for anywhere from 7 to 365 days and are sep-arated by a pain-free period of at least a month.

The length of each period or episode of cluster is often typical and they tend to be similar, but this is by no means the rule. The length of your period of cluster can change for no apparent reason. You can also swap from episodic to chronic cluster and back again.

I have had cluster headache since I was in my early 20s. It seems to be lasting longer now that I am older – is that normal?

The answer is 'Yes', but which bit is lasting longer? Each bout of pain during a period of cluster can last from 15 minutes up to 180 minutes. Each period of cluster can last for several weeks or months. Either way, though, any variation between these parameters is normal.

I used to get my cluster headache every spring but it now seems to come in the autumn as well. Should I be worried?

No, because the *frequency* and *periodicity* of your episodes of cluster can vary for any number of reasons. The IHS suggests that you must have a gap of at least one month between episodes. There is no limit to the number of episodes you can have. You just need to be tuned in to potential triggers to reduce the chance of an episode of cluster being set off.

> **My last bout of cluster headache just did not seem to want to stop. It usually lasts for only three months, so why did it seem to go on this time?**

That is difficult to say. The length of any period of cluster can vary. There is no particular reason for that bout to have been more prolonged but neither is there any reason why it should not last longer. Unfortunately, 10–15% of patients with cluster headache have chronic cluster headache without any break in symptoms.

It may be that there was one of several reasons within your diet or lifestyle that could have led to an extension of your symptoms on this occasion.

> **I have just been told that I have chronic cluster headache. What is the difference between chronic and episodic cluster headache?**

In simple terms, *episodic cluster headache* occurs in short but repeated bouts, but *chronic cluster headache* tends to occur for longer than a year without any breaks or with a break of less than one month.

> **In some attacks my headache lasts for 15 minutes but in other attacks it seems to last for an hour. Is that normal?**

Yes, the length of time the pain lasts can vary from attack to attack. It should last at least 15 minutes and no longer than 180 minutes to fulfil the IHS classification.

My best friend has just been told that she has SUNCT.
What is SUNCT?

SUNCT – the acronym for 'short-lasting unilateral neuralgiform headache attacks with conjunctival injection and tearing' – is a headache that lasts for only seconds and occurs between 3 and 240 times every day. The eye on the affected side tends to go very red and may water a lot. SUNCT is a type of headache that has become more recognised over the last decade but is very rare.

My cousin has cluster headache and his attacks last nearly
three hours but mine never last longer than half an hour.
Why is that?

How long the pain lasts can vary from person to person and from attack to attack. You are each showing duration consistent with the diagnosis of cluster headache. If the headache lasted for less than 15 minutes or longer than four hours the diagnosis might need to be reviewed according to the IHS criteria.

If it is very short-lived, it could be SUNCT; if it is longer than four hours, it might be migraine.

Sometimes I get my cluster pain four or five times in the day
and sometimes I don't get any for a day or two, when it seems
to come back with a vengeance. Why is that?

The pain of cluster headache can vary in frequency from day to day, as well as from episode to episode. The variability is unpredictable but this is normal. It is the unpredictability that can be frustrating!

In the same way, the severity and intensity of the pain can vary from attack to attack and from episode to episode. There will be times when the pain will be excruciating and potentially more difficult to treat.

My GP says that I have cluster migraine. What does he mean?

Cluster migraine is not a formal IHS diagnosis. It is difficult to know exactly what your GP means when using this phrase. It may be that he means your migraine headaches are coming together in groups or 'clusters' or it may mean that he thinks you actually have cluster headache.

Deciding which you have will depend on what other symptoms you experience at the time that you get your headache. If you get a red, watery eye and a runny or blocked nose and the pain is so severe you cannot keep still, it is likely that you have cluster headache. If you have a severe headache that makes you feel sick and you vomit and have to keep still or the pain gets worse when you move about, it is likely that you have migraine.

My son has cluster headache. I understand that it runs in families so can my daughter expect to get it?

Men are three to four times more likely than women to be affected with cluster headache. So your daughter could develop it but the risk is lower than if you had another son. Cluster headache may be inherited in 5% of cases.

My brother has cluster headache. Could I get it, too?

If you are male, the answer is yes. If you are female, it is less likely but still possible. Cluster headache is inherited in 5% of cases.

I've found that my cluster headache comes on after I've been out drinking with my mates. Will avoiding alcohol stop my next cluster attack from happening?

It is possible but by no means guaranteed that avoiding a bout of binge drinking could reduce the chance of triggering a period of cluster headache. If there are other potential triggers around, think about how these triggers come together. If moderating your volume of alcohol intake, especially at times of change, reduces the chance of cluster headache starting, it must be worth thinking about!

From what I've read on the internet, the pain I get seems like cluster headache but it only lasts for a few minutes and no longer than 30 minutes. Is it really cluster headache?

If you are female and the pain never lasts longer than 30 minutes, you get a red watery eye, and possibly a blocked or runny nose as well as some of the other cluster headache symptoms, you may have a condition called *paroxysmal hemicrania*.

The only way for your doctor to make a definite diagnosis is for you to take a course of indometacin. Paroxysmal hemicrania is called an 'indometacin-responsive' headache because the headache gets better with a course of indometacin. If your headache does not respond, it is not paroxysmal hemicrania but may be cluster headache.

You should see your GP to determine whether this is the case; she may suggest referring you to a neurologist or headache specialist for assessment, as it can be difficult to make a diagnosis. Sometimes it is just not possible to slot every headache into a 'diagnostic box'.

I seem to get bouts of pain for several weeks at a time. My specialist has told me I have paroxysmal hemicrania. My GP thought it was cluster headache, so how do they differ?

The main differences are that paroxysmal hemicrania is more common in women and always responds to indometacin. In many other ways, though, the symptoms associated with the headache are very similar.

4 | Other non-migraine headaches

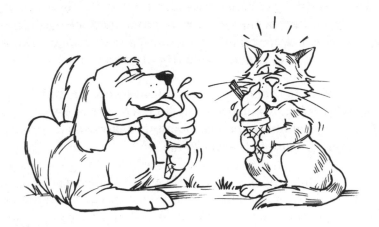

There are many 'primary' headaches that are not migraine, tension-type headaches or cluster headache. They are not very common but are included in this book so that, if you have these symptoms, you may be able to identify and diagnose the headache.

There are also headaches that are 'secondary' headache – the result of exposure to a substance or when that substance is removed.

STABS, JOLTS, EXERTIONAL AND OTHER SUDDEN ONSET OR SEVERE HEADACHES

My father has started waking in the night with a headache. It doesn't happen every night. The specialist has said it is hypnic headache. Can you tell me a bit more about it?

Hypnic headache used to be called an 'alarm clock' headache because it always wakes the person from sleep. Hypnic headache affects only people over the age of 50, occurs only during sleep and wakes the person with the headache. The headache tends to be dull, but may be severe in up to 20% of people. It can be associated with nausea or sensitivity to light or sound, but not both. There is none of the red eye or runny or blocked nose symptoms associated with cluster headache. The headache occurs at least 15 times each month and lasts for at least 15 minutes after waking, but no longer than 180 minutes.

I have been told that I have hypnic headache but I read somewhere that, if you get a new headache when you are older, you should be concerned about it. I have had a normal brain scan – should I be worried?

If your specialist feels that your headache fits into the 'hypnic headache' label and you have had a normal brain scan, there is no real cause for concern. It depends on how well your symptoms fit in the 'diagnostic box' and whether any change in your symptoms occurs over time.

I have heard of people having nerve pain and sciatica but what is neuralgia?

Neuralgia is a sharp, very short-lived, one-sided nerve pain. It can be described as like an electric shock or 'lancinating' (piercing), and lasts a few seconds with no symptoms between times. Different nerves can be affected and the pain is felt along the path of the nerve involved.

My aunt has trigeminal neuralgia. Can you tell me a bit about it?

Trigeminal neuralgia affects the cheek and chin most commonly and the pain never crosses the midline (the imaginary line that divides the left side of the body from the right). The pain is just like an electric shock and can be triggered by a variety of actions such as washing, shaving, talking, brushing teeth and other normal day-to-day activities. In any one person the attack follows the same pattern and is often precipitated by the same trigger spot.

Trigeminal neuralgia is not usually associated with a structural cause but, if it occurs on only one side of the face and is *always* on the same side, further assessment by a specialist might be a good idea.

My cousin has been getting these really sharp stabbing pains around his eye and temple. They are gone as soon as they have started. What sort of headache is it?

It is not always easy to answer this sort of question without gathering a lot more information. Assuming that your cousin has no other symptoms, such as nausea or a red watery eye that might suggest a different sort of headache, it may be a *primary stabbing headache*, previously known as 'ice-pick headache' or 'jabs and jolts'. The stabbing pain may move about the head, or swap sides.

Why do I get a headache when I am doing my aerobics class?

A headache can be triggered during exercise as a result of the exercise itself (a *benign exertional headache*), or as a result of dehydration or hypoglycaemia (low blood sugar) that can occur during exercise, and as such is a 'benign' headache. Exertional headache tends to occur more often at high altitude or during hot weather. The headache may last for at least five minutes and up to 48 hours after the exercise. More rarely, exertion can trigger a headache as a result of an underlying structural problem or anatomical abnormality – a secondary headache.

The first time such a headache occurs, a subarachnoid haemorrhage (SAH) needs to be excluded. This requires an emergency assessment, when a CT scan of the brain is done and, often, a lumbar puncture as well to look for red blood cells in the cerebrospinal fluid (CSF) that surrounds the brain.

There is more information on secondary headaches in Chapter 5.

I read a magazine article recently that indicates that it is
possible for a migraine to happen after having sex. Can
having sex really cause a headache?

Yes, it can, and is sometimes referred to as 'coital' or 'orgasmic headache'. The headache is often quite 'explosive' and of high impact when it occurs at orgasm. In someone with migraine the headache may be very like their usual migraine episode. This type of headache is usually benign but if it occurs for the first time, the person should see their doctor to make sure that the cause is not a subarachnoid haemorrhage.

A milder headache can occur before orgasm, which is of much lower impact and may be more like a tension-type headache.

I have, in the past, had a really bad migraine triggered
during intercourse. Should I be worried?

A severe, high-impact headache that occurs for the first time at orgasm is probably benign but you should see your doctor to make sure that it is not the result of a subarachnoid haemorrhage (SAH). If the headache recurs over time, it is more likely to be benign. If the headache is one-sided and is always on the same side, it might be wise for you to see your doctor to rule out an underlying structural cause, such as an aneurysm that might lead to a SAH.

MONOSODIUM GLUTAMATE, CARBON MONOXIDE, CAFFEINE AND OTHER STUFF

Headaches can occur for no apparent reason or as a result of exposure to a substance that causes or leads to the development of headache symptoms. These substances may be in prescribed medication and represent a side effect of that drug, or be in foods we eat or drinks we drink. As with any headache, not everyone is susceptible and there is no way of knowing if you are going to have a problem until you have been exposed to that substance. It may be that the headache starts as soon as you are exposed or you get the headache only when your exposure ends.

Why can't I ever eat a Chinese meal? It always gives me a migraine.

There is a headache associated with eating monosodium glutamate (MSG), which is found a lot in Chinese meals. The headache develops within one hour of eating the meal and settles within 72 hours.

The headache tends to be bilateral (affects both sides) and affects the forehead and temples. It is like migraine in that it is made worse with movement and tends to have a pulsating quality in people who have a history of migraine. It is often associated with other symptoms such as pressure in the chest or face, or burning sensations in the chest, neck or shoulders.

How can I tell if something I have eaten has caused my headache?

Food allergy is one thing, food sensitivity another – and either tends not to be a true trigger to migraine. The only way to know if a suspect food *does* trigger migraine is to exclude it from your diet for a month and then reintroduce it, keeping every other potential trigger the same. As you can imagine, this is not easy or even particularly realistic.

For more information about the effect of diet on your headache, have a look at Chapter 7.

Do chocolate and cheese trigger migraine?

Some people do feel that cheese triggers their migraine attack, and they avoid eating it. However, this effect has not been confirmed by scientific testing called 'challenge testing'. Tyramine, which was thought to be the reason for cheese triggering migraine attacks, was given to people who are 'cheese sensitive' and no attacks were triggered.

Chocolate contains tyramine and phenylethylamine, both of which were thought to be the potential trigger. A study using placebo (a 'dummy' ingredient) as well as active ingredients found that there was no difference in reaction between the people in the 'active' group and the placebo group.

These results tend to suggest that the answer to your question is 'No, chocolate and cheese do not trigger migraine'. It is also possible that the reason you always associate your migraine with these foods is that you have a craving for them during the warning or premonitory phase. This means that the attack was happening anyway and would have occurred even if you did not have the chocolate or the cheese. However, if you find that you tend to get a migraine every time you have them, they may be a true trigger for you. Everyone is different and rules are never absolute but the science suggests otherwise.

One of my friends has just been told that his headache could have been caused by a faulty boiler. Can that be true?

Yes, it is possible: a faulty boiler could lead to the build-up of carbon monoxide, which can cause headache symptoms. The headache often affects both sides of the head (bilateral) and tends to be continuous and of variable intensity. The severity of the headache may depend on the level of exposure to carbon monoxide. The headache develops within four to five days of exposure and settles within 72 hours after the exposure has ended – in your friend's case, once the boiler has been fixed.

The degree of exposure is assessed by measuring the level of carbon monoxide in the blood (the carboxyhaemoglobin level). The level of carboxyhaemoglobin determines the severity of the effect:

- Carboxyhaemoglobin level of 10–20%: mild headache only

- Carboxyhaemoglobin level of 20–30%: moderate, pulsating headache; irritability

- Carboxyhaemoglobin level of 30–40%: severe headache; nausea and vomiting; blurred vision

- Carboxyhaemoglobin level of more than 40%: tends to affect consciousness, so headache is not often complained of

It involves a simple blood test, ideally taken in the suspect environment, or very soon after leaving that environment. It needs to be taken very quickly because the levels start to fall as soon as you leave the area where the carbon monoxide is, and 50% has gone within four to five hours.

Why do I get a headache every time I have more than two or three glasses of wine?

If the headache has a direct cause and effect, it should start within three hours of drinking alcohol and will settle within 72 hours, according to the IHS criteria. The headache occurs on both sides of the head, tends to be across the forehead and temples, is pulsating and is made worse by movement.

If there is a delayed effect – the *hangover headache* – a migraine sufferer develops a headache after only a modest rather than an excessive amount of alcohol. The feature of the headache is as before. The headache develops after the blood alcohol level falls to zero and settles within 72 hours.

My neighbour told me that eating hot dogs can cause a headache. Is that really the case?

A *hot dog headache* is triggered by nitric oxide, which is found in cured meats – including 'hot dog' sausages. If you get migraine, you tend to get a migraine-type headache after eating a hot dog; if you have tension-type headache, you tend to get a tension-type headache; and if you normally have cluster headache, you get a cluster headache.

If your usual headache is migraine or tension type, the headache develops about five to six hours after exposure; if you have cluster headache, the headache develops after one to two hours.

A similar headache associated with nitrates is known as 'dynamite headache' or 'nitroglycerine headache'. This can be triggered by the use of nitrate sprays used to treat angina and was recognised in people who worked with munitions (dynamite).

My sister says that caffeine can cause my headaches but I don't see how this can be. I only get my headache at the weekend when I drink less coffee, rather than during the week when I drink it all day.

Caffeine does not actually cause headaches but the withdrawal or stopping of caffeine does. The resulting headache tends to occur on both sides and may have a pulsating feel. If you consume more than 200 mg of caffeine on a daily basis (see Tables 4.1 and 4.2) for at least two weeks, you may experience a headache within 24 hours of reducing or stopping taking caffeine. There is caffeine

Table 4.1 Caffeine content of drinks and foods

Item	Item size	Caffeine content
Coffee	150 ml (5 oz)	60–150 mg
Coffee, decaffeinated	150 ml (5 oz)	2–5 mg
Tea	150 ml (5 oz)	40–80 mg
Hot cocoa	150 ml (5 oz)	1–8 mg
Coca Cola	12 oz	64 mg
Diet Coca Cola	12 oz	45 mg
Dr Pepper	12 oz	61 mg
Pepsi Cola	12 oz	43 mg
Kit-Kat bar	1 bar, 47 g	5 mg
Chocolate brownie	1.25 oz	8 mg
Chocolate ice cream	50 g	2–5 mg
Milk chocolate	1 oz	1–15 mg
Special dark chocolate bar	1 bar, 41 g	31 mg
After Eight mint	2 pieces, 8 g	1.6 mg

Table 4.2 Caffeine content of over-the-counter painkillers

Name of preparation	Caffeine content
Alka-Seltzer XS	40 mg
Anadin Extra	45 mg
Anadin Maximum Strength	32 mg
Askit powders	110 mg
Boots Tension Headache Relief	30 mg
Hedex Extra	65 mg
Panadol Extra	65 mg
Phensic Dual Action	30 mg
Phensic Original	22 mg
Propain	50 mg
Solpadeine Plus	30 mg
Syndol	30 mg

in lots of products, not just drinks. There is caffeine in tea and coffee, and in lots of fizzy drinks, chocolate and over-the-counter painkillers.

For more information on how to raise your headache threshold and avoid a caffeine headache, see Chapter 7.

> **My cousin sometimes smokes cannabis and has found that he gets a headache a day or so later. Could cannabis cause his headaches?**

The use of cannabis can cause headache symptoms. This headache can be associated with a dry mouth, paraesthesiae (abnormal skin sensations, e.g. numbness), feeling warm and bloodshot eyes.

The headache itself tends to occur on both sides and is stabbing or pulsating, or is a feeling of pressure. It develops within 12 hours and settles within 72 hours.

I find that I can get a headache when I've been working at my PC all day. Can eye strain cause headache?

This is a controversial question, as some people will say 'Yes' and others will say 'No'. I suspect the reality is that it can – in some of the people some of the time, especially if other potential triggers co-exist. Posture can be as important a factor in this situation as anything else, so check your work station, and if you have not had a recent eye test, one might be worth considering.

If you need more information on optimising your work position, have a look at the Health and Safety Executive website (address in Appendix 1).

I have, once or twice, got a really nasty headache when I have had the air conditioning on in the car. I seem to be most sensitive when I have had it directed at my face. Is there anything I can do to stop it happening?

The only way to stop it happening is not turning on the air conditioning or at least directing it away from your face. As you have found, when the cold air passes through your nose or into your mouth, it can immediately cause a headache. The headache resolves quickly, usually within five minutes after turning off the air conditioning.

My sister can trigger a migraine when she eats really cold ice cream or sometimes when she crunches on ice cubes. I have never had this problem, though. Why is that?

Any cold stimulus has the capacity to cause a headache. The headache develops quickly and settles quickly. Ice cream, very cold drinks, crunching on ice cubes – all of them can do it. As with any headache, cold does not affect all of the people all of the time; it affects only some of the people some of the time!

5 | Recognising possibly more serious headaches

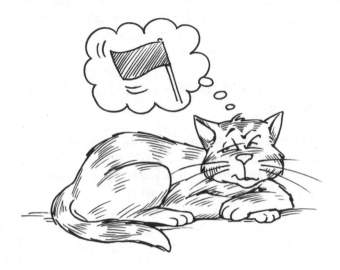

The words 'serious' or 'sinister' in connection with headaches means to most people making sure that there is not a brain tumour. In fact, a brain tumour is very rarely a cause of headache. The vast majority of headaches are what we call 'benign' – it is rare to find a serious or potentially sinister cause for a headache. We tend to be more concerned about a variety of other 'secondary' headaches that occur as a result of other medical conditions or specific structural abnormalities or injuries affecting parts of the brain and associated blood vessels, bones and surrounding structures.

Ruling out a serious headache is about taking a good history and trying to decide if this is a *primary* headache, such as migraine or cluster headache, or a *secondary* headache due to a brain tumour, stroke or other medical conditions.

My GP tells me that my headache symptoms are normal – they are not red flags. What are 'red flags'?

'Red flags' are the symptoms that may suggest to the doctor that your headache might be due to a more serious or 'sinister' underlying cause – a secondary rather than a primary headache. Sometimes these red flags have to be viewed in the context of your previous symptoms and sometimes they are important irrespective of your previous symptoms.

My headache always wakes me in the middle of the night. Should I be worried?

It is often said that a headache that causes you to wake up in the night, rather than a headache you become aware of when you wake in the night, is potentially serious or sinister. As with any 'rule' of this type, it is not absolute and needs to be considered in the context of the previous history of headache and any new symptoms that may be developing.

Cluster headache tends to occur during the night and will cause you to wake from your sleep. Migraine can also occur in the night, as does hypnic headache, and both will cause you to wake from your sleep. For more information on this, look at the 'specialist advice' section in Chapter 9.

I always get a really bad headache when I cough or sneeze. Should I do anything about it?

A headache made worse by coughing or sneezing is of no immediate concern. However, a headache that is *brought on* by coughing and sneezing and is very severe could suggest that there is an underlying structural lesion leading to a rise in cerebrospinal fluid (CSF) pressure within the skull – raised intracranial pressure – and hence causing the headache. When it occurs for the first time, it should be investigated to rule out a structural problem.

If you have had this symptom for months or even years, it is unlikely that there is any cause for concern. If it is something that is more recent and you get a severe headache that stops you dead in your tracks, I would suggest seeking advice from your GP. If you have had the symptom for some time but it is getting worse and now happens every time rather than some of the time, I would suggest seeing your GP for advice.

A *primary cough headache* is a benign headache that happens suddenly and lasts from one second to 30 minutes and is not the result of an underlying structural abnormality. It usually occurs on both sides (bilateral) and tends to affect people over the age of 40.

> *I am really embarrassed to go and see my GP because I*
> *have started to get headaches when I have sex. My sister says*
> *I should go, but I am not so sure. What should I do?*

Headaches can occur in a completely benign fashion in association with sexual activity, either during or before orgasm, and are referred to as 'primary orgasmic' or 'coital' headaches. When this occurs for the first time, it does need investigation and specialist referral to make absolutely sure that there is no structural cause for the headache – to make sure it is not a secondary headache. So you need to forget being embarrassed and go to see your GP so that you can be referred to a neurologist to be checked out.

Remember that doctors have seen and heard it all before!

> *I started with headaches a few weeks ago, and they seem to*
> *be getting worse very quickly. I don't want to waste my GP's*
> *time. What should I be looking out for?*

Headache is always difficult to assess in isolation and needs to be considered in the context of any other symptoms that you might have. If you do not normally get headache symptoms and your headaches seem to be progressing and getting worse over a few days or a few weeks, it would be sensible to go and chat to your GP to make sure there are no 'red flag' symptoms. Your GP will be able to examine you and make sure there is nothing serious or sinister to find, no physical signs or abnormality, anything that might suggest a secondary headache.

My father was walking along and complained of a severe headache on the back of his head. He couldn't carry on and a passer-by called for an ambulance. They insisted on taking him to A&E. Why was my father rushed to hospital when he got his headache?

A headache that comes on suddenly and dramatically may be due to a variety of potentially serious and significant structural causes – a secondary headache. The reason for taking him to hospital was to make sure he had not had a subarachnoid haemorrhage (SAH, bleeding onto the surface of the brain). A subarachnoid haemorrhage can occur as a result of:

- the rupture of an aneurysm (a ballooning and weakening of the wall of an artery) *or*

- an arteriovenous malformation (AVM, the structure of the arteries and veins is abnormal)

Because this can be fatal, a full and complete investigation and assessment is essential.

Headache is the only symptom in 12% of cases of SAH; it happens very suddenly, and is often described as 'being hit with a hammer'. It is often referred to as a 'thunderclap headache'. Neck stiffness can take up to three hours to develop, with varying changes in consciousness level occurring. SAH is often a cause of sudden death.

My mother got rushed in to hospital after complaining of a really bad headache, and they spent a lot of time trying to decide whether she should have a CT scan to diagnose a subarachnoid haemorrhage. Can you tell me why?

No test is done without good cause and a reasonable expectation of its providing the information needed to make a diagnosis. A CT scan can make a definite diagnosis of subarachnoid haemorrhage in 98% of cases if it is done within 12 hours of the headache starting. This falls to 93% at 24 hours, 76% at 48 hours and 58% at 5 days. These figures are from studies where expert radiologists read the scans and were able to interpret accurately quite subtle changes (with less skilled radiologists the pick-up rates are substantially lower).

Why did my father have to have a CT scan and a lumbar puncture to rule out a subarachnoid haemorrhage?

A lumbar puncture is done if the CT scan does not give a positive result despite symptoms that indicate SAH. The cerebrospinal fluid (CSF) pressure must be measured at the time that the lumbar puncture is done, to rule out the possibility of the procedure having caused any blood seen in the CSF. The CSF pressure will be raised if there has been a subarachnoid haemorrhage.

I have been told that I have migraine. During the last few attacks I have started getting pins and needles down my left arm. It starts in my hand and seems to move up my arm to my neck. Should I be worried?

Yes and no. It is always difficult to evaluate symptoms, as they need to be set in context. Provided that these sorts of sensory symptoms last for no longer than 60 minutes when they occur with a migraine headache, they are probably migrainous in their nature, rather than being due to a secondary cause. Sensory symptoms can extend into the headache phase of the attack but must settle before the headache does.

Symptoms that always occur on the same side may be due to an irritation of the nerve anywhere along its journey from the brain to its end. So, if your symptoms are always on the left side, they may be more likely to need investigating than if either or both sides are affected.

My brother says that his GP reckons that he had a transient ischaemic attack but what he described sounds like my migraine aura. What is the difference between them?

Symptoms of a transient ischaemic attack (TIA; a mini-stroke) can be very similar to those of a migraine aura. The main difference is usually how long they last and the fact that the symptoms of migraine aura are completely and totally reversible, usually over no more than one hour. If it is a TIA, it recovers completely within 24 hours but needs to be taken seriously because it indicates that there is probably something wrong with the blood supply to the brain.

What does the specialist mean by raised intracranial pressure? He was trying to explain something about why a headache can happen when you cough or strain.

The brain and spinal cord are surrounded by fluid called cerebrospinal fluid (CSF). Anything that affects the production, flow or absorption of CSF can lead to changes in intracranial pressure. A rise in pressure can occur with normal physical activities such as coughing or straining but, if there is a structural problem within the brain that affects the flow of CSF, this rise in pressure can be magnified and lead to a headache.

My grandmother has just been diagnosed with temporal arteritis. Can you tell me what that is?

Temporal arteritis is an inflammation in the temporal artery, causing pain that may be felt in the temple, over the forehead or the back of the head and occasionally more generally. The diagnosis may be made from a blood test, but if this is not conclusive, a biopsy of the temporal artery is needed (a tiny sample of the artery is taken for examination under a microscope). Early and prompt treatment is crucial to prevent complications such as blindness. Temporal arteritis is rare in anyone under the age of 55 and becomes more common as each decade passes.

My mother has been put on steroids for her temporal arteritis. How long will she have to be on them?

The response to steroids is swift, but treatment is medium term and is gradually reduced over months to years rather than weeks to months. Steroids have to be taken every day to be effective, and any dose reduction is usually monitored by a blood test. If there is any change in symptoms, following a dose reduction, she will need to increase the dose of steroids, usually for a few weeks before attempting another dose reduction. This is repeated in a step-wise fashion until the steroids have been stopped and all the symptoms have settled.

I think my friend should go to see her GP. She has been on the Pill for ages but has started getting flashing lights before her usual migraine starts. She says that the flashes last about an hour. She is not worried because her mum gets aura, but I read somewhere that if you have migraine you should not be on the Pill. What should I do?

You need to encourage her to see her GP to discuss her contraceptive options as, presumably, the last thing she wants is to get pregnant. She may have to stop the Pill she is currently taking, depending on which one it is.

There are two different female hormones: oestrogen and progesterone. If she has never had auras before, she should stop any Pill containing oestrogen. Anyone who has aura symptoms should not take a contraceptive Pill containing oestrogen, because of the increased risk of complications.

She can, however, carry on taking her Pill if it just contains progesterone.

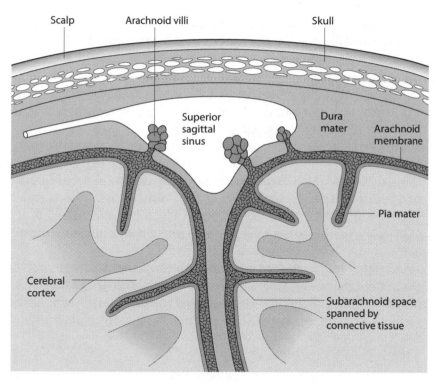

Figure 5.1 The brain and its protective meningeal layers, which may become inflamed as a result of infection.
(Adapted from *Target Migraine*, 2000, published by ABPI, London)

Dad has just started to get really bad headaches. He is 55 and smokes. The headaches are always on the same side. Should I make him go and see his GP?

You should encourage him to see his GP. Headaches starting in someone over 50 may be benign but the possibility of a structural or secondary cause needs to be ruled out. As a smoker, he is at risk of a variety of conditions that may cause headache symptoms. His GP will probably do some blood tests, arrange a chest x-ray and possibly refer him to a neurologist for a brain scan.

My cousin had what I thought was the flu, but he then got really bad headaches and was rushed into hospital. What caused his headache?

Any infection can cause headache symptoms, and without more information, or the results of his tests or investigations, I can't tell you exactly what caused his headache.

If the brain or its membranes become inflamed, you will develop a significant headache that is made worse by light and moving your head (neck stiffness). An inflammation of the brain would be an *encephalitis* and an inflammation of the lining of the brain is called *meningitis*. The meningeal membranes, which become inflamed, are in three layers: the dura mater, the arachnoid membrane and the pia mater; they can be clearly seen in Figure 5.1.

A variety of different viruses and bacteria can cause these sorts of infections, some of them more exotic than others. The viruses that cause some forms of encephalitis are associated with particular parts of the world, so a person's travel history is crucial in making a diagnosis.

What causes meningitis?

Meningitis is an inflammation of the meninges, which is the layer that covers the brain. Meningitis can be caused by a viral infection or a bacterial infection. (See Figure 5.1).

Meningococcal meningitis is the one that tends to make headlines. Other bacteria can cause meningitis and these include *Haemophilus influenzae* and *Streptococcus pneumoniae*. Meningitis, whatever the cause, is a serious condition that needs prompt diagnosis and aggressive treatment.

My uncle has a brain tumour. He started with a weakness of his hand that seemed to get worse and worse. Then his arm got weak, and then his foot started to go funny. What was happening?

Brain tumours may be *primary*, as a direct result of an abnormality within the brain itself, or *secondary*, due to the spread of cancerous cells from tumours in other parts of the body. The symptoms your uncle described suggest a tumour because the symptoms developed and progressed over a relatively short time – days and weeks rather than months and years. The symptoms that are seen or experienced are determined by which part of the brain is involved or damaged.

I always thought that you would get a headache if you had a brain tumour but my cousin has been diagnosed with a tumour and he never got a headache once. Why?

Headache is rarely an early symptom in patients with a brain tumour. No more than 20% of people with a brain tumour actually seek advice because of headache symptoms. The difficulty is that primary headaches can occur alongside secondary headaches and the skill of the doctor lies in deciding what the symptoms mean.

A brain tumour is usually recognised by the development of progressive physical symptoms – fits, sensory or motor changes (see the next answer for more information), sometimes emotional or psychological ones – and confirmed by a physical examination and further investigation.

My husband complained of a weakness of his arm. His GP thought that he had had a mini-stroke when he saw him because it seemed to have got better. Three days later my husband was admitted to hospital because the weakness came back and then got a lot worse. He also found he had difficulty walking. When he was seen in hospital the brain scan showed that he had a brain tumour. Should my GP have admitted him when he saw him the first time?

It is easy, in retrospect, to feel that a different choice should have been made. As the symptoms had improved by the time your GP saw your husband, a mini-stroke was the most reasonable and likely cause of your husband's symptoms initially. This is the difficulty with brain tumours. The diagnosis can only be made as *sensory* symptoms, such as pins and needles or numbness, or *motor* symptoms, such as weakness or paralysis, and *physical* signs, such as an inability to grip or use part of your body, develop and become obvious over time.

It is the speed with which symptoms develop and progress that raises the 'red flag' for the GP. I am sure there was no hesitation in admitting him to hospital when your GP reviewed your husband, as it became obvious that there was more going on.

6 | Who gets migraine and other headaches?

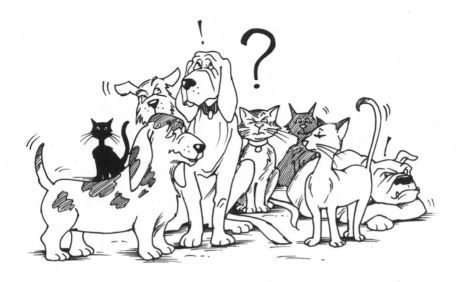

Headaches can affect anyone, at any time, for many different reasons and for no reason at all. Different people cope with headaches differently and different people perceive and experience pain differently.

HEREDITY AND GENDER

Both my partner and I suffer from migraines. Does this mean that our children will probably have them too?

Your children will be more likely to develop migraine than if neither one of you had migraine. A first-degree relative – a

Table 6.1 How many children suffer from migraine?

Author Country/year	Sample number	Age (years)	*Headache prevalence*			*Migraine prevalence*		
			Males	Females	Total	Males	Females	Total
Bille Sweden/1962	8,993	5–15						10.6
Linet USA/1984	10,132	12–29	90	95		5.3	14	
Mortimer UK/1992	1,083	3–11	40.6	36.9	38.9	4.1	2.9	3.7
Raieli Italy/1995	1,445	11–14	19.9	28.0	23.9	2.7	3.3	3.0
Sillanpaa Finland/1976–83	4,825	3		4.3				
		7				3.2	3.2	3.2
	3,784	13	79.8	84.2		8.1	15.1	

sibling or a child – is more likely to develop migraine than someone in the general population. There is no guarantee that they *will* develop migraine but, if the right triggers come together, they are more likely to have an attack. There is some evidence to suggest that this is more likely with migraine with aura.

There are various studies that have looked at just how many children suffer from migraine, and Table 6.1, which outlines findings from various countries, gives you a flavour of just how much of a problem it is.

I've heard that migraines are hereditary – both Mum and Dad get them, so is that why I get them as well?

The simple answer to that is 'Yes'. Studies have found that 50% of people with migraine know of a relative who has migraine, and as many as 90% have a first-degree relative (parent, sibling, child) who has migraine.

***My sister told me that an article she read says that
migraines get better as you get older. I hope this is right!***

Generally, migraine does become less common as you get older.
Headaches can still occur but they may not be due to migraine.
The type of headache may change with age: for example, tension-type
headache due to neck problems, temporal arteritis or an increase in
migraine due to the menopause.

***Is it true that people with certain personalities are more
likely to get migraine?***

Anyone can get headache and no one particular personality is
more likely to get headache or migraine than any other. *But*
some people cope better with pain than others. Some people are tuned
in to possible triggers or things that push their migraine threshold
down, so they are more likely to get migraine. Self-awareness, knowing and understanding how things affect you, and insight,
recognising that things need to change, can be relevant to managing
and coping with headaches.

For more information about raising your headache threshold, look
at Chapter 7.

***As children, my brother got migraine and I didn't; now that
we are teenagers, I get migraine and my brother doesn't.
Any idea why?***

The facts seem to be that boys are affected more commonly than
girls, but in adulthood, women are more commonly affected than
men. Why this is so is less clear but, as the change occurs at or around
the time of puberty, there is an assumption that the female hormone
oestrogen is the likely reason. (See also the next answer.)

Why are more women affected with migraine than men?

There is no doubt that more women are affected by migraine than men. It is assumed that, because this shift occurs around the time of puberty, oestrogen is the reason for this change.

There is evidence that some women get a migraine headache at the start of their period and that this is associated with the size and rate of the fall in oestrogen levels. In addition, a significant proportion of women who have migraine, especially the type without aura, tend to become migraine-free during pregnancy, a time when oestrogen levels are stable.

Is it true that men are more likely than women to have cluster headache?

Yes, that does seem to be the case. Women can get cluster headache but it is much more common in men. Nevertheless, it is a very rare condition, only 0.5% of the UK population being affected.

I understand that migraines are more common in women and cluster headaches are more common in men. Do other types of headache show a difference between the sexes?

Statistics indicate that:

- *tension-type headache* affects both men and women, but 90% of women are affected compared with 70% of men

- *cluster headache* affects more men than women in a ratio of 3:1

- *coital headache* can occur at the start of sexual activity or at orgasm; it is more common in men but does occur in women as well, the ratio is about 4:1

- *paroxysmal hemicrania* is more common in women than in men in a ratio of 3:1

Are there any racial differences between who gets migraine and who does not?

Ethnic and cultural differences in people who get migraine headaches and those who don't may be related to perception and coping strategies. Nevertheless, 'white' (Caucasian) people seem to be affected more than Afro-Caribbean and Asian people.

My mother suffered quite badly with migraines and I get them, too. Is migraine inherited?

Familial hemiplegic migraine is a migraine that runs in families (hence the term 'familial') and causes paralysis down one side (hemiplegic). It is a genetic condition that has been linked to specific genes on particular chromosomes and is transmitted as an autosomal dominant characteristic. 'Autosomal dominant' means that you need only one parent to have the gene for you to inherit/develop the condition.

The gene in the case of familial hemiplegic migraine is located on chromosome 19. The abnormality is present on the cell membrane, which controls the passage of calcium, sodium and potassium in and out of the cell. When the relevant gene is present on chromosome 19, the passage of calcium through the membrane is abnormal; this alters the 'conductivity' of the nerve cell, which predisposes to migraine.

For those of you who feel like trying to understand a little more, read on . . .

There are three 'loci', points, on chromosomes – FHM1, FHM2 and FHM3 – each associated with a specific chromosome and gene. The defect associated with locus FHM1 is on chromosome 19, specifically 19p13. The gene has been identified as CACNA1A. The defect associated with locus FHM2 is on chromosome 1, specifically 1q21-q23. The gene has been identified as ATP1A2. The defect associated with locus FHM3 is on chromosome 2, specifically 2q24. The gene has been identified as SCN1A.

These defects are associated with a variety of *channelopathies*. A channelopathy is a condition or disease that involves the ion channels in cell membranes and how 'ions' (calcium, sodium and potassium) move across cell membranes. If these ions do not move freely and normally, the cell does not perform its normal healthy function and disease results.

The CACNA1A gene is associated with P/Q-type calcium channels, the ATP1A2 gene is associated with a sodium/potassium transportation mechanism and the SCN1A is associated with a sodium channel protein.

OTHER FACTORS BEHIND HEADACHES

Are there any particular medical conditions that might mean I am more likely to get a headache?

Headache is a very common symptom and may occur coincidentally with other disease processes or be directly related to those processes. For example, poorly controlled diabetes or an overactive thyroid gland may lead to an increase in headache symptoms. Anxiety and depression are not uncommon in migraine sufferers – but which comes first? Any infection from the common cold to meningitis may be associated with headache symptoms.

There is a very definite association between stroke and migraine, migraine with aura being a much greater risk factor than migraine without aura. In some instances a stroke may lead to migraine symptoms developing.

For more information on understanding risk factors, look in Chapter 7.

***At my first visit to the specialist, he asked me how old I am.
How is that relevant?***

Age is important because certain headaches are associated with particular times of life. People at different ages can have an increased risk of developing medical conditions that may give rise to headache symptoms.

***I started getting migraines a few years ago, when I was 22.
Is how old I am likely to affect my migraine?***

Anyone can get migraine, irrespective of age. Migraine tends to occur for the first time when you are in your 20s to 40s. It should occur less often once you get into your 50s and 60s but it can still occur.

You can see some of the statistics in Figure 6.1.

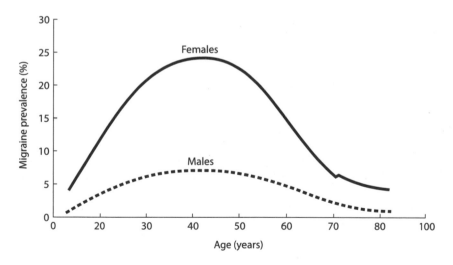

Figure 6.1 The prevalence of migraine according to age
and gender (from data by Lipton and colleagues 1993, 2000).

For information on raising your headache threshold, look at Chapter 7.

I hardly ever used to get headaches until I moved to another job. Can the job I do affect my headache?

Your job may affect your headache, if you let it. Posture, meal patterns, fluid intake and stress may all push your migraine threshold down. Poor posture, certain lighting conditions or situations, prolonged periods of driving and working shifts may all contribute to headache symptoms. It is not the job itself that may contribute to headache symptoms but how you manage and cope on a day-to-day basis.

7 | How can I help myself?

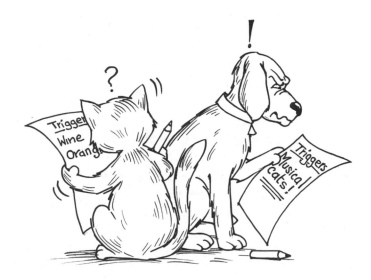

Migraine can leave you feeling as if you are not in control of your life. It may feel as though your migraine decides what you can and cannot do rather than your deciding what you want to do. Being aware of how different aspects of your diet and lifestyle (see Table 7.1) can affect your migraine threshold will help you take back control.

UNDERSTANDING YOUR MIGRAINE THRESHOLD

My mum and dad both have migraines. I've heard that migraines are hereditary, so just how much can I help myself to have fewer attacks?

Yes, a family history of migraine does mean that you are more likely to develop migraine at some time in your life. There is no

Table 7.1 Diet and lifestyle strategies to keep your headache threshold as high as possible

DIET

Try to eat regularly:
- every 4 hours in the day
- a break no longer than 12 hours overnight
- be extra vigilant when travelling, having the weekend lie-in, change in shifts, social functions if eating late

Avoid known food triggers, if you have any

Avoid processed sugars and junk foods as much as possible:
- eat regularly, eat healthily
- eat low glycaemic index foods if possible

Stay well hydrated:
- 2 litres of water every day, more in hot weather
- reduce caffeine intake as much as possible
- avoid fizzy drinks as much as possible (think about caffeine and artificial sweeteners)

STRESS

Try to put yourself first at least once every day:
- start with 5 minutes and build up to 30 minutes
- relax any way you can

Try to take regular exercise

Try to plan ahead if you expect a busy day or week:
- remember to ask for help or support
- people will help if you ask them

Try to maintain a regular sleep pattern:
- too much or too little sleep can trigger headaches

Modify your work environment:
- check your work posture
- get your work station checked
- think about lighting
- remember to take regular breaks

At times of hormonal change try to be more in control of other triggers to keep your headache threshold high guarantee that attacks *will* develop but an awareness of potential triggers will reduce the chance of attacks developing if these triggers do come together and lower your migraine threshold. This chapter discusses ways to help you modify your headache threshold and take control of your headache symptoms.

I heard part of a programme discussing migraine and missed the beginning. Can you explain what is meant by the phrase 'migraine threshold'?

Anyone has the potential to have a migraine. Your 'migraine threshold' is the point below which a migraine attack becomes inevitable. The higher your threshold, the less likely you are to have a migraine. Being aware of potential factors or triggers in your life and being in control of them will reduce the chance of your threshold being pushed so low that an attack becomes inevitable. This is different for everyone – Figure 7.1 illustrates this.

I'd like to try to avoid setting off a migraine if possible. What brings on a migraine?

This is not an easy question to answer, because in reality it is impossible to say. A migraine can happen at any time. All you need is the right mix of triggers together at the right time – the challenge being that the mix will vary every time. The attack happens when all those factors come together and your migraine threshold is finally reached.

I am trying to work out what triggers my migraine but don't know how to go about it. Please help!

It is not an easy thing to do, as there is unlikely to be a cut-and-dried answer. You will have to keep a diary but before doing so you need to decide what factors you want to consider. Do you want to think about meal patterns, fluid intake, your menstrual periods or

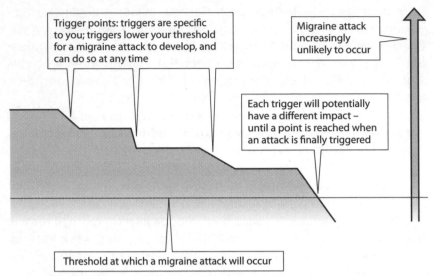

Figure 7.1 Example of migraine threshold and how triggers can affect it.

specific foods? What you have to remember is that triggers tend to work in combination rather than in isolation, and you may find it difficult to find a consistent pattern.

> *I was listening to something on the radio recently and they kept talking about common triggers but did not really say what they are. Can you tell what they meant by common triggers?*

In reality the phrase probably means different things to different people. A *trigger* is something that increases the chance of a migraine attack happening. 'Common' triggers are generally regarded as things such as chocolate, cheese and red wine (there is more information about these later in this chapter). Other 'common' triggers in my experience include things such as irregular eating patterns, irregular or erratic sleep patterns, dehydration, too much caffeine or even caffeine withdrawal; all these can lead to a lowered migraine threshold. Other factors include stress and sometimes back or neck problems associated with muscle spasm, which can lower your migraine threshold and increase the chance of an attack being triggered.

I keep reading about common triggers. I have tried avoiding them but it doesn't seem to make any difference. Why is this?

Triggers tend to be very personal and vary from person to person. What seems to trigger an attack in one person may never trigger an attack in someone else. Moreover, the effect or impact of a trigger may vary in the same person from day to day, week to week and attack to attack. The steps you take to reduce the chance of an attack developing may well change the effect that any one trigger has on you at that time. Figure 7.2 outlines how triggers can affect your migraine threshold.

The other day I was so busy that I couldn't stop for lunch. Later I got a really persistent migraine. Are the two related?

The simple answer is 'Yes, possibly'. To understand why this is, we need to think about where your migraine threshold is – look at Figure 7.2. If you go without eating for more than 4 hours in the daytime or 12 hours overnight, you could push your migraine threshold so low that an attack is triggered. On this occasion, missing lunch took you from point D to E and an attack was triggered.

I've heard that some people with migraine find that certain foods will set off a migraine. What sort of food can trigger migraine?

Any food can potentially trigger migraine in some of the people, some of the time! The difficulty is deciding which food, in which

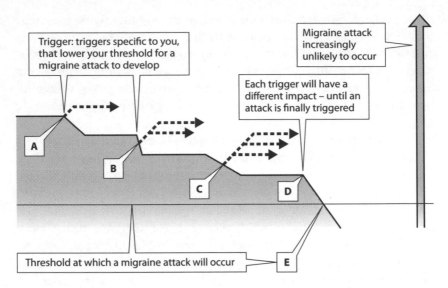

Figure 7.2 How triggers affect your migraine threshold.
A: Point at which a trigger may push your threshold down, OR you can make a positive change that will push your threshold up. **B**: Point at which a trigger or triggers can push your threshold down, OR you can make a series of changes that can raise your threshold; the effect can and will vary.
C: Different triggers can and will affect you in different ways; different combinations of triggers tend to have differing effects at different times, as will the steps you take to raise your threshold. **D**: Point at which an attack is almost inevitable. **E**: Point at which a migraine attack will happen.

people and when. Some people find that a particular food will always trigger an attack all of the time. In some people a particular food will trigger an attack some of the time. If the food trigger is inconsistent, this usually means that the most relevant factor is where your migraine threshold is, rather than the food itself. (There is more information on this aspect in Chapter 4.)

A friend gave me a list of foods I should avoid to prevent my migraine attacks from happening. There are so many things listed I think I'd rather risk the migraine!

In many ways you are probably right to be cautious about avoiding so many different foods. A healthy and varied diet is much more likely to reduce the chance of migraines developing than a restricted and faddy diet. Eating regular meals and having healthy snacks is more likely to raise your migraine threshold. If a specific food triggers your attacks, you will probably have worked this out by now. If you have not identified anything, it is unlikely that one food triggers your attacks all of the time.

I have cut out chocolate, cheese and alcohol but I still get migraines. Why?

Chocolate, cheese and alcohol are rarely true migraine triggers that have a direct cause and effect when it comes to migraine. They may actually represent cravings at the start of the attack, rather than a cause. You may be at point A (see Figure 7.2) rather than point D. (There is more information about this aspect in Chapter 4.)

Triggers are very personal and can vary from attack to attack as well as from person to person and from time to time. The main variable is your migraine threshold at the time that you are exposed to a potential trigger. The other variable is what you do at a point in time or in response to a series of events that may push your migraine threshold down to modify the potential effect of any one trigger.

I've read that scientists now say chocolate isn't a trigger. I can't believe this, as I get migraine if I eat chocolate when I'm feeling a bit under par but not when I'm feeling fit. Surely they've got it wrong?

In some people specific foods may have a direct cause and effect but it is also possible that a craving for a particular food occurs during the premonitory or warning phase of a migraine. There is a perception that the chocolate caused the attack but, in fact, the attack was happening anyway, so the chocolate is not a direct cause. It may be that in your case it has a partial effect and pushes your threshold down so that, if you are feeling under par, your migraine is triggered … or it may be that feeling under par is what really triggered the migraine. Figure 7.3 reminds you of the phases and patterns of a migraine attack.

There is more information about food factors in Chapter 4.

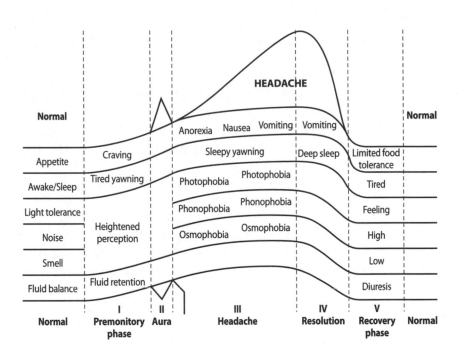

Figure 7.3 The phases and patterns of a migraine attack.
(Adapted from JN Blau, 1992, 'Migraine: theories of pathogenesis',
Lancet, vol.339: 1202–7)

Cheese and oranges don't seem to affect me but red wine and red meat do. Is there a connection?

Everyone is different and what is important is that you recognise the factors that are relevant to you and take control of those specific triggers as you find them. It may be that you can manage to eat the red meat or drink the red wine separately but not have them together or that you can have them without triggering a migraine when your migraine threshold is high. (There is more information about this aspect in Chapter 4.)

Why is it that sometimes I can eat cheese with no problems and other times I have a migraine?

Triggers tend to work in combination rather than in isolation. You could try analysing what other constants exist when you eat cheese and it seems to trigger a migraine. A little bit of detective work might allow you to find out a few more dos and don'ts and so find a way of keeping your migraine threshold up enough to have cheese. Whenever you have a migraine after eating cheese, try to remember what else preceded the attack: you may find that there is another factor involved.

I understand that everyone is affected differently but how can I decide which triggers are relevant to me?

If you look back at Figure 7.2, you can see that at different points (A, B, etc.) a particular trigger or food could have an effect on your migraine threshold. If you are at point D or E, it is more likely that a particular food will trigger your attack as it pushes your threshold down to the point at which an attack becomes inevitable.

If you want to see whether a food is going to cause you problems, I suggest you avoid that food – and that food only – for a period of four to six weeks. You should then reintroduce that food and see if your attacks return. The food may directly trigger the attack or could lead to an increase in frequency of attacks. This avoidance of a food is helpful only if all other triggers stay stable, and that is often impossible to achieve.

Triggers aren't just about food but are also about things such as irregular meals, too much caffeine, not enough water and changes in sleep patterns. Triggers tend to work in combination rather than in isolation. A food may be part of a broader, complex mix, making specifics difficult to identify. So look at your life generally to see if you can discover a connection between your migraines and other possible triggers. It might take a bit of time but you'll be doing something positive to help yourself.

I often have a migraine on the day before a party that I've been looking forward to, so I end up not going. How can I stop this from happening?

This is quite a common experience. Getting excited about an event can have the same effect on your migraine threshold as getting anxious and upset about it. Getting and feeling in control can be difficult in this situation. Making a special effort to control all other aspects of your day can keep your threshold a little higher and reduce the chance of an attack developing. It is about pushing your threshold from C or D back to B or A (see Figure 7.2).

I often seem to have a migraine at the weekend. Why is this?

This 'relaxation' headache is not unusual for some people. It is often the case if you have a busy and potentially stressful existence. The need to get through the week is such that the migraine attack never develops until it is safe for you to 'allow' it to. (See Table 7.1 for more advice.)

Why do I always seem to get a migraine on the first few days of my holiday?

A 'relaxation' headache is not uncommon, and the start of a holiday is a period of relaxation. In part it is due to a variety of factors that lead to a change in your migraine threshold. The build-up to a holiday is often a busy and difficult time. Travelling from your home to your holiday destination is also associated with its own hassles and stresses, including missed and skipped meals, loss of sleep and dehydration. Taking all these factors together, it is not surprising that a migraine might happen. Think about the bits you can control, so that the rest will have less of an effect on your migraine threshold.

Why do I always seem to get more migraines when I am working nights rather than a day shift?

Working nights is likely to be associated with a more erratic eating pattern as well as a degree of sleep deprivation and probably an element of dehydration, too. All these elements will tend to push your migraine threshold down and increase the chance of a migraine attack being triggered.

Why is it that I often get a migraine when I am going out to the theatre after work, especially if I don't get time to eat beforehand?

That is likely to be a mix of the stress associated with getting to the theatre in time, dehydration for a similar reason combined with prolonging the period without food. You could try to reduce some of the pressure by leaving work early so that you are less stressed and have time for a meal before you go out. If you can't do that, try to have a light snack before you go out. You need to think about what you have to do to nudge your migraine threshold up and reduce the risk of a migraine attack developing at some time in the evening.

Can changes in the weather be a trigger? I seem to get a
migraine when a thunderstorm is approaching and
sometimes just before it snows.

Changes in barometric pressure associated with changes in the weather have been found to cause an increase in headaches and migraine. Humidity is another factor along with bright, especially flickering, sunlight and cold winds.

My cousin says that she often gets a migraine when she has
to work in an office with fluorescent lighting. Is there a
connection?

Lighting is always difficult to evaluate but the brightness of fluorescent lighting may cause a degree of glare that could lower her migraine threshold. And the flicker of a fluorescent light can cause migraine in some people.

Sometimes being sick makes me feel better. Does this mean
that the migraine was caused by something I ate?

No, it does not. Vomiting is a recognised symptom of the migraine attack, and the onset of vomiting during an attack shows that the attack is progressing. As you have found, having been sick, you often start to get better.

I have four or five triggers but I find it frustrating always
making sure that they don't clash too much. What practical
steps can I take?

It may be that you don't need to avoid all of them at the same time. You may find that one or two of them together are OK. Working out which combination you can cope with is very much trial and error, and may depend on exactly where your threshold is and how sensitive you are to particular triggers. Keeping a diary, perhaps using diary cards, might help you in your detective work. (For information about diary cards, see the 'Specialist nurse' section in Chapter 10.)

My main triggers seem to be cheese, chocolate, red wine, oranges and being very tired but sometimes I can eat or drink these items with no ill-effects whereas at other times they'll trigger a migraine. Is there a 'threshold' to these triggers?

There is a 'threshold' for your migraine but not specifically a threshold for your triggers. Each trigger has the ability to push your migraine threshold down but the extent to which it does so is variable and unpredictable. Your recognised trigger will have an effect sometimes rather than all the time, because it will take a different mix each time to have the same overall effect on your migraine threshold. (There is more information about this aspect of food in Chapter 4.)

I've never had two migraines in the same week that were 'set off' by the same trigger. Does this mean that the attack makes me briefly immune to its trigger?

No, not really. Migraine attacks can happen at any time: the lower your threshold, the more likely an attack is to be triggered. Triggers rarely work in isolation, so any trigger can lead to an attack at any time, and are rarely consistent in how long they last.

I find that I'm more likely to have a migraine if I've been under a lot of pressure at work. Is there a connection?

Stress is a very potent trigger and can often have a significant effect on your migraine threshold, even in isolation. It can magnify the effect of other triggers, so that things that do not usually trigger attacks may become more likely to do so. It's hard to get rid of all pressure at work but knowing that it can be a factor in triggering a migraine should help you to avoid anything else that might contribute to lowering your migraine threshold. Take control of the things that you can control so that the factors you cannot control are less likely to push your threshold down.

> **Stress seems to be a common cause of my migraine but part of my problem is worrying when I will get another attack. What can I do?**

Stress tends to be a very potent trigger and can readily push your migraine threshold down. If you are going through a phase of frequent attacks, it is not surprising that you become anxious about another attack developing. If you try to take positive steps to raise your migraine threshold, you are less likely to get an attack and will move into a more positive cycle. I tend to offer the following advice:

- Eat regular meals, keep your sugar levels steady
- Avoid known trigger foods and drinks
- Avoid prolonged fasting, avoid hunger
- Ensure adequate fluid intake, avoid thirst
- Be consistent in your sleep habits
- Avoid stress where possible, relieve stress when you can
- Keep your attack threshold high by avoiding multiple triggers
- Don't be afraid to ask for advice and help

See Table 7.1 at the beginning of this chapter for more suggestions.

UNDERSTANDING YOUR FOOD – GLYCAEMIC INDEX AND WHAT IT MEANS

I have been reading in newspapers and magazines about low GI and high GI foods. Can you explain what it means?

GI stands for glycaemic index, and is a calculation of how quickly a food is broken down into its constituent parts, specifically looking at glucose, by the digestive system. A high GI food is broken down quickly and a low GI food is broken down more slowly.

Why is GI measured?

Measuring GI helps you understand more about the food you eat. Foods that are low GI tend to be healthier because they contain starch as well as sugar and are rich in fibre, vitamins, minerals and antioxidants. Low GI foods tend to leave you feeling fuller, so you are less likely to snack between meals; because they are broken down more slowly, they tend to keep your sugar levels more even.

Understanding GI is not just about specific foods but also about what happens when those foods come together on your plate.

What sorts of foods are low GI?

Low GI foods are those that are rated below 55. They include cereals such as oatmeal, bran and bran flakes, fresh pasta, basmati rice and all types of fresh fruit, including oranges, apples and grapefruit as well as pure fruit juices.

What foods are high GI?

Sugar is rated as 100, and other foods that are high GI are certain breads such as baguettes, white bread and bagels; cereals such as cornflakes, frosted flakes, sugar puffs and honey and nut cornflakes as well as Healthy Living Sultana bran.

Are there any foods that come in the middle when it comes to GI?

Yes, there are: cereals such as fruit muesli, fruit and fibre breakfast cereal and whole wheat muesli; breads such as pitta bread, multi-grain loaf and multi-grain batch bread; also new potatoes and sweet potatoes.

How can I find out more about GI foods and diets?

There are many books available now that give lots of information on GI diets and preparing food the GI way. All you need is a good bookshop or library.

How can I plan a healthy meal?

This is about getting the right balance of the different food groups on your plate. You need about 50–55% carbohydrate, 15% protein and 35% fat to give you what you need to keep your body healthy. Remember that it needs to be 'good' fats not 'bad' fats to keep you healthy.

How you prepare and cook food is also important; for example, mashed potatoes and jacket potatoes are higher GI than new potatoes. Always undercook vegetables, pasta and rice, as cooking starts to break down foods and speeds up the digestive process – making the food higher in its GI value. Home-made soups are much lower GI than tinned or prepared soups.

Is there anything I can do to make my meal more low GI?

Yes, you can. Protein, fats and fibre all slow down the digestive process, so a meal that has a mix of all the food groups tends to produce a slower release of sugar into the blood stream and hence a lower GI meal. You need healthy fats, not fats that could raise your cholesterol; remember that a lot of 'healthy eating, low fat' prepared foods are often high in sugar, so read the packaging and see what the sugar levels are like.

UNDERSTANDING RISK FACTORS

What does my GP mean when she says I need to minimise my risk factors?

The sorts of things your GP is concerned about are:

- Do you smoke?
- How much alcohol do you drink?
- Do you take regular exercise?
- What is your diet like?
  - Is it low in fat?
  - Is it high in fibre?
- Are you overweight?
- Is your blood pressure normal?
- What is your cholesterol?
  - Do you have the right balance of good and bad cholesterol?
- What is your blood sugar?

These are all aspects of our life that may contribute to the development of disease. If you are overweight, you are at a greater risk of developing high blood pressure or diabetes. High blood pressure or diabetes may increase your chance of a heart attack – an event we would all prefer to avoid.

Minimising your risk factors is making sure that your lifestyle is as healthy as possible so that you reduce the chance of developing a disease that may be potentially life-threatening.

I have migraine and want to go on the Pill. Why is my GP so keen for me to stop smoking?

Your GP wants to minimise the risk to you of going on the Pill. Migraine is associated with an increased risk of stroke, and going on the Pill increases your risk of stroke. The biggest risk of stroke is smoking, so your GP simply wants to make your going on the Pill as safe as possible from a medical risk perspective. (See Chapter 15 for more information.)

I am taking a triptan for my migraine but my GP says I have to stop it until my blood pressure is under control. Why?

A raised blood pressure can lead to a variety of medical conditions, one of which is a heart attack or stroke. Triptans work by causing blood vessels to constrict and narrow. If your blood pressure remains untreated, this could lead to vessel damage – which is magnified when you take your triptan to treat your migraine and could theoretically cause a heart attack or stroke.

Your GP wants to minimise the risk of this happening. Getting your blood pressure under control minimises your risk of these other conditions developing and allows you to treat your migraine effectively and safely again.

I have a strong family history of heart attack, and a lot of my family get migraine. What sort of risk factors should I think about?

You need to think about your cholesterol levels, especially your balance of good and bad cholesterol. If you smoke, you should stop; if you are overweight, you should think about trying to lose some weight. These steps will reduce your risk of both heart attack (a potential risk associated with your family history) and stroke (a potential risk associated with your migraine).

You might want to think about a low GI diet, which is said to aid weight loss, as is regular exercise. These are all things that can reduce the risk to you of a heart attack happening.

OVER-THE-COUNTER OPTIONS FOR TREATMENT

I have started to get some headaches, and wondered if there is anything that I can buy that might help?

Most people with headache and migraine use over-the-counter (OTC – without a prescription) medication very effectively. We all have headaches from time to time, and using medication every now and again is not a problem. Different drugs work differently: depending on the headache you have, most simple painkillers work well, especially if taken early enough.

For more advice on how to treat your headache, look at Chapter 11.

I tried taking aspirin for my headache but it did not help very much. There are so many different brands, how can I decide what else to try?

Different brands often have different amounts of aspirin in the tablet, and may have other drugs or compounds in the tablet. The mix may include paracetamol or codeine as well as some caffeine. The only way to find out which one works for you is to try it, but you have to make sure that you are treating the right headache with the right option.

You may need to seek advice from your GP to determine which headache you have and/or what treatment is best. Chapters 2, 3, 4 and 5 discuss diagnosis and Chapters 11 and 12 have information about treatment.

Does it make any difference if I buy painkillers from the local chemist or the supermarket?

No, it doesn't. If you have a painkiller that works well for your headache, where you buy it will not make any difference. What you need to think about is making sure that you only have a headache now and again.

For information about developing medication overuse headache (MOH), look at Chapter 3.

I have tried various drugs from the chemist but I just seem to vomit them back. Is there anything else I could buy?

There are some over-the-counter (OTC) options that contain drugs to help with the nausea and vomiting. Migraleve contains an anti-nausea drug as well as paracetamol to treat migraine. You can also buy a drug called domperidone over the counter, which will help the nausea and get the painkiller absorbed more quickly.

For more advice on acute treatment for your headache, look at Chapter 11.

Do things like 4head work?

My reply is: does it work for you? It can help some people ease their headache symptoms. If you find that it helps, then fine; others find that a cold flannel can work just as well.

I have just heard that there is a new drug I can get from my pharmacist without a prescription. I think it is called Imigran. What is it?

It is indeed Imigran but it is not in fact a new drug. It has been available for over 10 years but until recently has been available only on prescription from your GP. It is one of a group or class of drugs called triptans. There are seven different triptans and Imigran (generic name sumatriptan) is one of them. You will need to speak to your pharmacist, who will ask you some questions to check that it is a suitable drug for you to use.

For more information about triptans, look in Chapter 11.

8 | Complementary therapies

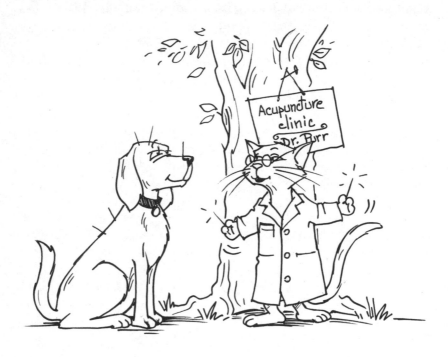

'Complementary therapy' suggests an approach that is used *as well as* or to support more traditional medical treatment. 'Alternative therapy' suggests an approach that is used *instead of* rather than in support of more traditional types of care. Complementary is the phrase that best reflects the point at which these therapies should be considered. It should not be an 'either/or' but an 'as well as'. Physical therapies, such as aromatherapy, rarely do harm and, if nothing else, often allow you to have a 'time out' from what may be a full and busy day, week or month. Think about your migraine threshold and all the things that you could do to raise that threshold.

Herbal remedies are often seen as natural and therefore must be safe. This is not always so, as there are documented incidents when people have become ill, or even died, after taking herbal remedies, whether Eastern or Western in their source. Many factors are relevant, including where the plants were grown, when they were harvested and how pure the final product is.

Remember that few complementary therapies are available on the NHS, and you will have to pay for them yourself. When considering trying out a complementary therapy, ask the practitioner as many questions as you want or need before committing yourself. You need to be sure that they have all the relevant qualifications, are registered with a professional body and have appropriate insurance. With therapies that are regulated by law, there should be no problems because you can check with the relevant body that the therapist is registered with them. Be wary of anyone who promises to cure your headaches for ever or recommends that you use a therapy without first discussing it with your GP. Although some doctors are sceptical about the value of complementary therapies, they are usually happy for you to try something else if traditional medicine hasn't really been able to help. But your doctor knows about your overall health and is better equipped to advise you about any possibly doubtful aspects.

Everyone is looking for a 'cure' for their headaches and a huge industry has evolved in the complementary therapy area. None of these therapies will specifically treat your migraine but the range of approaches has the potential to modify or improve pain and your response to pain; it is a preventative rather than an acute treatment. Complementary therapies are not free and you need to be just as informed about using them and choosing your therapist as you would about anything else you invest in.

There is value in a therapy only if it 'works' and the only way to be certain of that is to undertake a clinical trial to assess the effectiveness of any therapy. The quality of research in the area of complementary therapy is variable and sometimes difficult to evaluate. In this chapter I have tried to offer an objective view of the data and evidence available.

ACUPUNCTURE AND ACUPRESSURE

My neighbour has suggested that I try acupuncture.
What actually is acupuncture?

Acupuncture is a Chinese traditional therapy where very fine needles are inserted at specific points around the body. It is based on the premise that these points lie on 'meridians' along which the body energy flows. This body energy, or 'chi', is a balance between the positive and negative – the 'yin' and 'yang'. When this energy or chi goes out of balance, the body experiences symptoms and these can be corrected by using the needles to release the blockage. Different points relate to specific body organs and are used to treat specific conditions. The needles are left in for 30 minutes.

I am not sure I fancy the thought of needles being stuck in me. How many will be used, and will I feel them?

You will not really feel the needles, as they are very fine indeed. You can expect between four and ten needles to be used. There will probably be some sensation connected with the needles but some practitioners believe that this shows that the acupuncture point is being stimulated.

Even if I accept that having needles stuck in me won't hurt, how safe is acupuncture?

Although there is no formal system for reporting problems experienced with acupuncture, it does seem to be a safe form of treatment. Serious problems are usually associated with poor practice, the most common being forgotten needles and transient low blood pressure; less common problems include localised bruising or a flare-up of symptoms.

Who can do acupuncture? If it's just anyone, I don't think I want to risk it!

Anyone can be an acupuncturist, provided they complete the necessary training. Many different health-care professionals have trained to give acupuncture as part of their role, including doctors, nurses, midwives and physiotherapists, but an acupuncturist does not have to have a medical background.

Doctors and nurses have to train for years. How long do acupuncturists have to train?

Professional acupuncturists train for up to three or four years full-time and may have a university degree on completion, or complete further training in Chinese herbalism. Medical acupuncturists undergo fewer training hours, often during weekend courses, and learn a small range of techniques only.

If acupuncturists have all this training, do they have to be registered as well?

The training for acupuncture is independently accredited by the British Acupuncture Accreditation Board. Ordinary practitioners of acupuncture are registered with and regulated by the British Acupuncture Council (BAcC).

Physiotherapists who also do acupuncture are regulated by the Acupuncture Association of Chartered Physiotherapists (AACP).

Doctors, who will already have completed a medical degree and other forms of postgraduate training, can complete a Certificate of Basic Competence and a Diploma of Medical Acupuncture via the British Medical Acupuncture Society.

Can acupuncture help my migraine?

Acupuncture is thought to stimulate the release of a range of chemicals (neurotransmitters) called endorphins, encephalins and serotonin. Endorphins and encephalins are opioid peptides and are the body's natural painkillers. It may be that the release of these chemicals during the treatment relieves the pain of the migraine headache. Acupuncture can also help treat nausea and thus can relieve this symptom during the migraine attack.

Acupuncture may help your migraine symptoms or may reduce the total number of attacks you experience: the only way you will know is by trying it out. The benefit may be short-lived or permanent; if it is only short-lived, the effect can be sustained by repeating the treatment from time to time, perhaps every four to six weeks.

Can acupuncture help my tension-type headache?

Acupuncture can be of benefit for a range of pain conditions and so it may well ease or relieve your headache. The only way to find out is to try a course of perhaps four treatments. If four treatments have no effect, though, it is probably not worth pursuing further.

Acupuncture sounds as though it's worth trying. How can I find an acupuncturist?

The best and simplest starting point is the British Acupuncture Council (their contact details are given in Appendix 1). They should be able to give you names of practitioners in your area. Or you could ask your GP, who might already know of someone locally.

How can I tell if acupuncture is making a difference to my migraine?

It depends on what you mean by 'difference'. It may be that acupuncture can reduce the severity of symptoms during the acute attack, or shorten the length of the attack, or make the attack easier to treat or reduce the total number of headache days experienced. You need to decide which of these options best reflects what you want or expect from the course of treatment. If you are lucky, it may improve or modify one or all of these areas. You won't know until you try, as there is no way of predicting if acupuncture can help you.

How many acupuncture sessions am I likely to need to make a difference?

That is quite difficult to answer. If you notice no change after four sessions, it is unlikely to make a difference. If it *is* making a difference, you may need as few as six or as many as twelve sessions to produce an improvement.

I found that the last time I had some acupuncture it settled my headache down really well but they seemed to creep back in again after a few months. Do I need to keep it 'topped up'?

If it has worked well but the symptoms come back after you have completed a course of treatment, you may find that having a session every four to six weeks is all you need to do to keep things under control. Talk to the acupuncturist about this.

What is the difference between acupressure and acupuncture?

Whereas acupuncture uses needles, acupressure uses finger pressure at specific points along the body to treat pain, including headache, and a variety of conditions associated with stress. If you hate the idea of needles, this is certainly worth a try.

Can I apply acupressure myself?

There is no reason why not. We often apply pressure instinctively when we experience pain by massaging an area that feels sore or uncomfortable. All you need to do is learn the points that you can use if you feel a headache building.

OSTEOPATHY AND CHIROPRACTIC

From what I've heard of osteopathy and chiropractic, they seem very similar. How are they different?

Osteopathy and chiropractic are both forms of manipulation therapies. Chiropractic was founded by Daniel D Palmer and osteopathy was founded by Andrew Taylor Still. They are very similar therapies, working with bones, muscles, tendons and ligaments to treat problems with structure and function but practitioners of chiropractic believe that many health problems are caused by the spine being out of alignment.

Are osteopathy and chiropractic safe?

The most common unwanted effects tend to be mild pain or discomfort at the site of manipulation, slight headache or fatigue; the vast majority resolve within 24 hours. Risk factors need to be evaluated before treatment is commenced to minimise the chance of more serious complications occurring.

The most serious events are associated with neck manipulation and include stroke and injury to the spinal cord. They are very rare, though, and statistics range from 1 in 20,000 to 1 in a million neck manipulations. If you are considering trying either technique, talk to the practitioner frankly about any reservations you might have.

What is osteopathy? My cousin says it has helped her headaches.

Osteopathy is a form of therapy based on the idea that the musculo-skeletal system is at the root of many disorders and conditions. Osteopaths work by manipulating your muscles, joints and tendons. Some employ a variety of techniques using limbs to make 'levered thrusts' or functional techniques using gentle but prolonged pull and rotation to release muscle tension and ease symptoms.

Some also use techniques called cranial osteopathy or cranio-sacral therapy, in which they gently manipulate the bones of the skull and sacrum to correct symptoms.

In the UK, osteopaths are regulated by the General Osteopathic Council, established by two Acts of Parliament passed in the mid-1990s. They complete a full-time four-year course and achieve a BSc degree (BOst).

I hate relying on drugs to control my headaches. Might a course of osteopathy help?

Headache is a pain condition and osteopathy can help ease pain symptoms. Headache symptoms may be triggered from neck or back problems, leading to muscle spasm and hence headache. Osteopathy may be able to relieve neck and back problems and therefore the muscle spasm. This in turn will tend to raise the threshold for triggering symptoms of a headache, the headache being either a tension-type headache or a migraine.

I'd like to try osteopathy to see if it helps. How can I find an osteopath?

The best source of information will be the regulatory body, the General Osteopathic Council (contact details in Appendix 1). Or your GP might know of an osteopath who practises in your area. Remember, though, that your GP may not be happy to suggest a local therapist if one is not personally known to them.

If osteopathy does not help me, could or should I try seeing a chiropractor?

It is possible that, for you, one treatment will work better than the other, and you are unlikely to come to harm by trying either or both. It may be that the slightly different philosophies and approaches to treatment will produce a more positive outcome. The only way to find out is to try the other if the first does not seem to help you in the way that you wish or expect.

Are chiropractors registered and regulated in the same way as osteopaths?

Yes, they are. Chiropractors are regulated by two Acts of Parliament passed in the mid-1990s that established the General Chiropractic Council. They complete a full-time four- or five-year course and achieve a BSc degree in human sciences and chiropractic. There is also a postgraduate year of training that results in a diploma in chiropractic. All chiropractors are able to apply for membership of the College of Chiropractors, which has a regional network for continuing professional development.

What can I expect during a course of chiropractic treatment?

Chiropractors use a short, sharp motion or 'high-velocity thrust' applied to the spine and may also use a range of soft-tissue manipulation techniques that are gentler. McTimoney chiropractic has its own range of techniques, with less emphasis on high-velocity thrusts.

Each session lasts between 15 and 30 minutes, and up to six sessions are needed. The first few sessions tend to be given at fairly short intervals, becoming less frequent with time.

I'd like to try chiropractic. How can I find a chiropractor near me?

The best source of information will be the General Chiropractic Council (contact details in Appendix 1). Or your GP might know of a chiropractor who practises in your area. Remember, though, that your GP may not be happy to suggest a local therapist if one is not personally known to them.

HOMOEOPATHY

My cousin has suggested I try homoeopathy rather than the migraine tablets I take. What is it, and could it help me?

Homoeopathy is a form of therapy developed on the principle of treating like with like; a very diluted amount of a substance is given that, undiluted, would normally reproduce the symptoms of the illness but when given in such minute quantities produces a 'cure'. The homoeopath is treating you as a person, rather than the migraine itself. A qualified homoeopath will tailor the treatment to you as an individual, so it is better to seek advice from a qualified therapist, rather than try something you have bought yourself.

There are five homoeopathic hospitals in the UK within the NHS. As with any NHS service, you need a GP referral to be seen. The hospitals are scattered around the country, so they are not necessarily readily accessible to everyone.

ALEXANDER TECHNIQUE

I saw a magazine article that suggested that the Alexander Technique can help with migraines. Is this so?

If posture and work position have an effect on how your headaches develop, the Alexander Technique may help you. It is a way of bringing your posture back to the optimal and heightening your awareness in order to make good posture and movement the norm. It is about balance. It is a technique that may take months or years to perfect.

To find a teacher of the Alexander Technique, contact their headquarters (address in Appendix 1).

MASSAGE THERAPIES

A work colleague keeps saying how wonderful reflexology has been for her. What is reflexology?

Reflexology is one of the massage therapies. Parts of the foot are reckoned to correspond to areas of the body; if any part of the foot is tender, it is massaged gently to release 'toxins' that are believed to be the cause. As a result, there is an improvement in general health or in the symptoms associated with that particular part of the body.

Reflexology seems to work for some people with different conditions. Should I try it for my headaches?

Reflexology is unlikely to cause you any harm and may be of some benefit. If you try two or three sessions, you will be able to see whether it makes any difference. Note, though, that any therapy you try is about breaking the headache cycle you are in and is not likely to prevent all your headaches for ever.

Is seeing a reflexologist likely to help my migraine?

A foot massage is certainly a relaxing experience and any opportunity for a bit of 'me time' in a busy day or week will be able to push up your migraine threshold and reduce the chance of a migraine attack being triggered.

Several of my friends have found aromatherapy helpful in their busy lives. Can you tell me a bit about it?

A romatherapy was first described in 1928 by a French chemist Gattefossé working in his family perfumery business. In 1964 Dr Jean Valnet published a paper in the journal *Aromathérapie* showing that he could successfully treat specific medical and psychiatric disorders using essential oils. (Essential oils in their natural form are much more effective than any synthetic substitute.)

Essential oils are absorbed through the skin when used in massage treatment. Different oils are absorbed at different rates and have three modes of action: on a pharmacological, a physiological and a psychological level.

If you know that certain smells or scents can trigger your migraine, be sure to mention it to the therapist, and remember to check that he or she is using unscented base oil.

Lots of people seem to like aromatherapy. Is it safe?

M assage is, in large part, safe. However, it should avoided on an area of skin that is damaged or burnt, or on a limb if there has been a deep vein thrombosis (DVT). There is no evidence to suggest that cancer can be spread by massage but it is best to avoid treatment directly over the cancer site.

The essential oils in aromatherapy are used externally and in low concentration. Nevertheless, some should be avoided in certain medical or physiological conditions. This means that it is vital that any massage therapist is fully aware of any and all co-existing medical conditions.

Who can do aromatherapy or massage?

At present, anyone can be an aromatherapist – there is no statutory regulation of the therapy. However, many physiotherapists as well as specifically trained massage and aromatherapists can use aromatherapy and massage. A range of health-care professionals can also be trained in using these approaches to support patients. The Aromatherapy Consortium is working towards voluntary regulation of aromatherapy and already has developed training and competence standards for its members.

How would aromatherapy help me and my headaches?

Different oils have different effects. For example:

- chamomile, bergamot, sandalwood, lavender and sweet marjoram have a sedative effect on the nervous system

- jasmine, peppermint, basil, clove and ylang ylang have a stimulating effect on the nervous system

Oils can have an effect at a physiological level but another effect at a psychological level. Ylang ylang and jasmine can be nerve stimulants but have a soothing and relaxing effect as well.

What oils are recommended for headache symptoms?

These essential oils can be used for massage, as a compress and as a vapour to ease headache symptoms:

- chamomile (German and Roman), lavender (spike and true) and mint (peppermint and spearmint) are probably more effective and tend to be more readily available

- less commonly available, and possibly less effective, are citronella, cumin, eucalyptus (blue gum and peppermint), grapefruit, lemongrass, sweet marjoram, rose (cabbage and damask), rosemary, rosewood, sage (clary and Spanish), thyme and violet

Are there any oils that are more effective for migraine than for 'ordinary' headache?

Essential oils suggested for migraine alone should be used as a compress; they include angelica, lemon balm, French basil, coriander, linden, clary sage, valerian and yarrow. Essential oils suggested for headache as well as migraine include chamomile, citronella, lavender, sweet marjoram and mint.

The most effective, and possibly the most readily available, is true lavender (*Lavandula angustifolia*).

What can I expect from a massage session?

First, you will need to remove all your clothes, but will usually be given a towel to cover yourself with. You will be asked to lie on a couch in a warm room, often with soothing music being played. The massage will often focus on parts of the body that feel sore or tender, using a range of techniques of gentle stroking, firm pressure, deep massage and light slaps or karate chops. Oil is used to aid the process of the massage and aromatherapy oils may be added.

In the interests of practicality and speed there are times when just the hands or feet are rubbed or the neck or shoulder may be massaged · through clothes.

I am thinking about trying aromatherapy. How can I find a reliable therapist?

The best source of information would be the British Complementary Medicine Association. It has developed training and competence standards, and has a panel that regularly reviews its members. You might also try the Aromatherapy Consortium. Contact details for both are in Appendix 1.

HYPNOSIS

Hypnotherapy helped my husband stop smoking. Would it help me prevent migraines?

It could help you learn how to control some of the factors that may have an effect on your migraine threshold. Different people find different therapies work for them and you have little to lose in trying hypnotherapy.

How does hypnosis work? My brother found it helpful for coping with pain after he was injured in an accident.

Hypnosis is a way of giving you coping strategies while you are in a relaxed state, or what is called an altered level of consciousness. These coping strategies work at a subconscious level to help you manage your pain. Relaxation and self-suggestion may bring about behavioural and emotional changes.

Changing your behaviour is about modifying or altering how you respond to pain, as this may change how the pain progresses and builds or settles. Your emotional state also has the ability to affect how you feel and experience pain. Anything that can modify your behavioural or emotional response has the potential to raise your headache threshold.

Hypnosis is unlikely to be helpful after a single session, though. It takes time to translate the subconscious feeling of control into a conscious level of self-hypnosis that will help you control the pain of your headache when it is developing. If you decide to give hypnosis a try, you should use a qualified, able and competent therapist (see the next answer).

What training do doctors have before being able to do hypnotherapy?

There are basic, intermediate and advanced courses for doctors and dentists as well as regular scientific meetings. These are run by the British Society of Medical and Dental Hypnosis.

Is hypnotherapy safe? I wouldn't want to try it if there might be problems afterwards.

Hypnotherapy is, by and large, safe, unless there is a pre-existing significant psychiatric or psychological problem that might be affected or modified.

If I decide to try hypnosis, how do I find a reputable hypnotherapist?

The British Psychological Society will be able to suggest a reputable hypnotherapist, who will be a Chartered Psychologist who works within a recognised code of conduct. Contact details of the Society are in Appendix 1. You could also contact the National Council of Hypnotherapy (details also in Appendix 1).

YOGA AND MEDITATION

Quite a few people have suggested that I ought to give yoga a try. It seems a bit faddy to me; can you tell me a bit about it?

Yoga comes from India and is a way of achieving relaxation by controlling the body and the mind. It is the ability to learn relaxation techniques and meditation that are of value to the headache sufferer. The core principles of healthy food and regular meal patterns are also helpful in raising your headache or migraine threshold.

Today's lives tend to be full and busy, and many people find yoga calming and relaxing. Any opportunity to have some protected time that will ease the stresses and pressures will be of benefit. You have nothing to lose and possibly a lot to gain by giving it a go.

Can meditation help my headache?

Meditation can help headache, chronic pain, anxiety and stress. It is a way of promoting both physical and emotional relaxation. Making it part of the day can help raise the migraine threshold and reduce the chance of an attack being triggered.

You need to consider meditation as a way of focusing your attention away from the pain. The focus may be an image, sound, word or phrase; returning to this while you are meditating or experiencing the start of a headache helps prevent it from developing.

I have a lot of neck and head pain. Is relaxation and meditation likely to help?

Pain, especially chronic (long-term) pain, can be helped by relaxation techniques, and learning the art of meditation helps you learn how to relax. Relaxing and learning how to change negative stress to positive stress can only be a good thing in raising your migraine threshold or preventing your threshold from being pushed down.

BIOFEEDBACK

I was reading in the paper that, if you make your hand warm, your headache will get better. Does that actually work?

There have been some studies which suggest that, if you warm the hand opposite to the side the headache is, the headache will get better. With training, you can use *biofeedback* to raise the temperature of the hand and ease the headache symptoms, rather than putting your hand in hot water.

For more about biofeedback, see the next two answers.

What is biofeedback, and can it help tension-type headache?

It is possible to measure the amount of spasm in your neck muscles using something called EMG – electromyography. Biofeedback is about making you aware of how tense your muscles are so that you can relax them. With this technique you learn to recognise how the muscles feel using a biofeedback machine and how to relax the muscles at will – thereby easing or preventing the tension-type headache. Eventually you will be able to achieve this relaxation without the machine.

Can biofeedback do something to stop my migraine happening?

Some studies have shown that a migraine sufferer can learn how to constrict their temporal artery, which becomes dilated at the start of the migraine attack. By constricting the artery, the attack can be aborted.

It is possible that using biofeedback to relax neck and shoulder muscles may help in raising your migraine threshold and thus prevent a migraine attack from being triggered. Biofeedback has the potential to help and will not cause any harm.

FEVERFEW

My cousin swears by feverfew leaves, which she has every day. I find them rather bitter, though. Can I get them in tablet form?

Feverfew (*Tanacetum parthenium*) is available as the pure leaf or leaf extract, both of them in capsule form. The pure leaf form is taken three times a day and the leaf extract just once daily.

How can I be sure I am taking the right amount of feverfew?

Research suggests that 100 mg of leaf extract, once daily, should be taken with food. You should take it for three months to see if there is a reduction in headache days. If there is no effect at that dose, it is probably not going to help.

For how long should I take the feverfew?

Feverfew is used as a preventative drug, and these are usually taken for three months to see if there is any response. If at the end of three months there has been an improvement, it is reasonable to take it for a total of six months before stopping it. If the attacks come back, you can always start taking it again.

Are there any side effects I can expect from using feverfew?

Mouth ulcers tend to be the main side effect experienced with feverfew. You may experience soreness or inflammation of the mouth and even a loss of taste. Other side effects include a bitter taste in the mouth, indigestion, diarrhoea, and possibly nausea and/or vomiting.

Should I talk to my GP before trying feverfew?

It is not essential to see your GP but it might be worth checking that your blood pressure is normal. You should not use feverfew if you are on the contraceptive Pill, or are pregnant or breast feeding.

MINERALS, VITAMINS AND SUPPLEMENTS

Someone in my local health-food shop suggested that I try magnesium. Does magnesium work?

Magnesium was found to be effective in two out of three trials in reducing the frequency of migraine but side effects were relatively high. Diarrhoea affected nearly 20% of people and irritation of the stomach affected nearly 5%.

What dose of magnesium should I take?

The dose of magnesium used in trials looking at migraine prevention was 300 mg a day.

If I find that magnesium works for me, how long should I take it?

Using magnesium in this way is about migraine prevention, so you should try it for three months and see if there is a reduction in headache days at the end of that time.

Any preventative drug should be taken for three months to assess whether there is any reduction in headache frequency. If there is no significant change, it should be stopped. If there is some improvement, continue taking it for a maximum of six months and then stop it. The aim is to break the cycle of headache days – there is no treatment that will be able to stop them completely.

Another customer in the health-food shop was buying riboflavin for her headache. What is riboflavin? Can it help my migraine?

Riboflavin, vitamin B_2, is a co-enzyme that is involved in energy production in the muscle cells of the body. (An enzyme is a protein that controls chemical reactions that occur in the body, and a co-enzyme is a substance that is essential for enzymes to work and do the job they were designed for.)

The results of trials using riboflavin have suggested that it is effective in reducing the number of migraines experienced.

If I decide to try riboflavin, what dose would I need to take?

The recommended dose is 400 mg a day. You may notice some benefit after a few weeks but the maximum potential effect will be achieved after three months of daily treatment. The most dramatic side effect is that it turns urine bright yellow. The only other side effects that have been documented are diarrhoea and polyuria (passing a lot of urine).

Someone suggested that butterbur could help my migraine. Can you tell me a bit about it?

Butterbur must be used in the form of purified root extract. It has been shown to reduce the frequency of migraine attacks by more than 50% when taken by adults for four months at a dose of 75 mg twice a day. It has been used with good effect in children aged 6 to 9 years at a dose of 25 mg twice daily and in adolescents aged 10 to 17 years at a dose of 50 mg twice daily.

Could co-enzyme Q10 work in reducing the number of migraines I get?

Co-enzyme Q10, if taken, is used as a preventative drug. A small study found that co-enzyme Q10 at a dose of 150 mg a day reduced the number of migraine days by more than 50%.

REIKI

I was reading an article recently about complementary therapies, and it mentioned Reiki. What is Reiki?

Reiki is a Japanese word meaning 'universal energy' or 'universal life energy'. It is a system of natural healing in which the Reiki practitioner places their hands over the body of someone who is lying down, fully clothed, and relaxed. The healing is said to occur at any level, be it physical, mental, emotional or spiritual.

Reiki sounds a bit way out. Is it safe?

It is said that Reiki is gentle and can be used for a wide variety of conditions in many different settings. Although there is no scientific evidence supporting its healing claims, it involves relaxation, which might help you and certainly won't do any harm.

If I decide to try it, what can I expect from a Reiki session?

You should wear comfortable clothes and will be encouraged to either sit or lie down. The practitioner will have a light and gentle touch. You may feel heat, tingling, coolness or throbbing sensations under the hand as it moves around your body, or you may feel nothing at all. At the end of the session, which can last up to an hour, you should be left with a feeling of well-being and relaxation, or may come away feeling energised. Everyone is different.

9 | Who can help me?

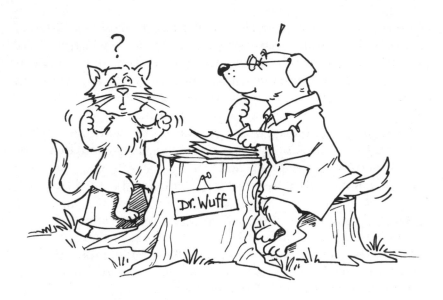

Several health professionals are available to help you. Initially, the local pharmacist can offer information and advice about dealing with quite a wide range of problems, and will know when to advise you to consult your GP for investigation and treatment. This includes coping with headaches.

Your GP will be able to assess your headache and offer appropriate advice and assessment in the first instance or may ask other members of the Primary Health Care Team to offer you advice or support as you try to get back in control of your headache symptoms. If your GP feels unable to help or improve things, a referral to a GP with a special interest (GPwSI) or neurologist might be appropriate. If you are very lucky, you may also get access to a Specialist Headache Nurse.

THE COMMUNITY PHARMACIST

I have started to get the occasional headache. Is the local pharmacist likely to be able to help?

Your pharmacist will be able to offer advice about the different sorts of painkillers that you can buy 'over the counter' (OTC; without a prescription), which may help you improve or control your headache symptoms. Your pharmacist will also have some awareness of the risks of taking too many painkillers and how this might lead to your developing a medication overuse headache.

A triptan, sumatriptan, is now available from your pharmacist, once they have determined that it is the right drug to use to treat your migraine and safe for you to take.

For more information on acute treatment, see Chapter 11.

When I first started taking painkillers for my headaches, they helped, but nowadays I seem to keep taking them just to stop the headache from coming back. The pharmacist felt that provided I did not take more than the prescribed dose there should not be a problem. Please help!

It sounds as if you might be taking too many painkillers. This results in a medication overuse headache where the painkillers seem to drive the headache rather than stop it. You need to stop all the painkillers. This is not always easy and you may well need help from your GP. Your GP may help you himself or refer you to a specialist headache centre.

My pharmacist tells me that I might be making my headaches worse by taking so many painkillers. What does she mean?

There is some evidence that taking painkillers to treat headache symptoms on most days, even if it's just a single dose, can lead to a medication overuse headache. In crude terms, the brain's pain receptors are being kept 'on' rather than being switched off by the tablets. The more often you take the painkillers, the more headaches you get, and the more painkillers you seem to need. The headache just never seems to go away completely.

I have tried lots of different tablets for my headache. Should I go back to the pharmacist or is it time to see my GP?

I suspect the time has come to see your GP. Treating headache is about making sure you know what your headache is before you can find the right treatment for it. There are ways of managing your headache without taking any tablets at all. If you have tried too many tablets or are taking them too often, you may need your GP's help to stop using them. If there are any worrying symptoms, your GP may want to refer you to a specialist.

My GP has said that I can buy ibuprofen and domperidone from the local chemist without a prescription. My GP wrote down what doses to take but the pharmacist has said that they are too big. Who is right?

They are both right, in terms of the guidelines they work within. Drugs that can be purchased over the counter are not always available at the same sort of doses as your GP can prescribe for you. Buying drugs 'over the counter' can be a cheaper option than paying a full prescription charge, which may be why your GP suggested that you do this.

For more information about drug dosages, see Chapter 11 on acute treatments.

What is a 'prescription pre-payment certificate'? It was something that the pharmacy assistant mentioned.

If you pay for your prescriptions, you could buy a prescription 'season ticket': you pay a fixed sum in advance, and that covers you for all NHS prescriptions for a certain period. This scheme is worth it if you have 6 or more items in four months or 15 or more items in a year. At the time of writing (2006) the cost was £6.65 per item or £34.65 for four months or £95.30 for a year. You can apply for this pre-payment certificate on form FP95, which is available at most chemist/pharmacist shops and main post offices or from your Primary Care Trust.

THE GENERAL PRACTITIONER (GP)

The pharmacist has recommended that I see my GP about my migraines. How can she help me with them?

Your GP can help but not all GPs have a particular interest in headache problems. She can listen to what you say, and will often be able to make a formal diagnosis as well as suggesting various treatment options. If your GP does not feel able to help, she will be able to refer you to a specialist with an interest in headache.

If my GP refers me to someone else, is it likely to be to a neurologist?

Yes, your GP may refer you to a neurologist. If he does, you should ideally see a neurologist with an interest in headache problems. A specialist centre supported by specialist headache nurses would be even better. Your GP will refer you if he has worries or concerns about your headache and associated symptoms or he is having difficulty controlling your headache.

My GP says that she might refer me to a specialist about my headaches. Can she refer me to the specialist I want to see?

The answer to that question is not as straightforward as it should be. If there is a specialist service local to where you are, the referral is straightforward and the time it takes will simply reflect the local waiting time and capacity. However, if there isn't a specialist headache service already contracted to provide a service for your Primary Care Trust (PCT), the PCT may not agree to fund a referral out of your local area. If there is a local neurologist but the service offered is not a specialist one, again the PCT may choose not to fund the referral.

The challenge in the NHS is limited resources and how these are spent. There are no barriers if you can afford to go privately or your local health provider is able and willing to fund the referral as an NHS referral.

> *I feel that my GP isn't being very helpful. Although I've told him that the headache of my migraine starts in the night when I'm asleep, he just tells me to take painkillers when I feel the attack starting! What can I do, as it's quite severe when I wake up?*

In absolute terms your GP is correct, as painkillers will not stop your migraine from starting if you take them at bedtime – before the attack starts. You need to wait until the warning symptoms begin or the headache begins for them to work. You need to think about possible reasons why the migraine starts in the night. Are you dehydrated? Should you think about having a light snack before going to bed? Have you got over-stressed? The higher your migraine threshold is, the less likely an attack is to start.

There is no realistic way of knowing if your attack is going to start in the absence of any symptoms. If you take a tablet just in case a headache is going to happen, you could potentially take a painkiller every night – which will inevitably lead to a medication overuse headache.

If, however, you have warning or premonitory symptoms before you go to bed, it makes sense to take a first-step treatment such as ibuprofen at the right dose.

For more advice about how to treat your migraine, see Chapter 11. If you want to raise your migraine threshold, look at Chapter 7.

I have been to see my GP several times about my migraines but nothing I've tried seems to work. What can I do to find a better treatment?

There are a lot of options and everyone is different so you need to keep trying until you find a mix or combination that works. Your GP will be able to offer you a variety of different drugs: anti-inflammatories, anti-emetics and triptans. You can take these in many different combinations at the start of the attack and repeat the dose of anti-inflammatories through the next 24 hours. If you get a lot of nausea or vomiting, the anti-emetic can be repeated as well to improve the effectiveness of other treatments.

It is a question of trial and error. It would be great if you could find the right treatment first time but that rarely happens. Managing migraine is not just about taking tablets – it's about lots of other things as well. Remember to eat and drink regularly, treat your attack early and give your treatment a chance to work.

How can I get my GP to take my migraine seriously? I get the feeling that she thinks I'm making a fuss about nothing.

You can help your GP by thinking about what you want to say before you go. Write it all down so that you don't forget. If possible, make a double appointment to see your GP. Having more time will take the pressure off both of you. You'll be able to get your message across by making sure you have told your GP everything you want her to know.

My GP says that I have medication overuse headache and must stop taking the painkillers completely. I'm going to need some time off work to do this; will she be able to give me a sick note for it?

Your GP will be able to give you a sick note if you feel that you need time off work to succeed. Your GP, family, friends and work colleagues will need to work together and support you so that you can successfully stop your painkillers. (Dealing with medication overuse headache is discussed in Chapter 13.)

> **Can I ask my GP to give me a different triptan? I've been reading about the zolmitriptan nasal spray and, as I feel sick early on, think it might work better for me.**

If you feel you want to try something different, certainly ask your GP. Remember to explain why you want to try something else. A nasal spray may well be a good idea, especially as you get nausea early in your attack. There are two different nasal sprays available: one is zolmitriptan and the other is sumatriptan. If one does not work well for you, the other is certainly worth a try.

> **I have been on several different websites and read about eletriptan but my GP has not heard about it. Why is this?**

If you live in England or Wales, the reason for this will be that, when eletriptan was launched for use on prescription, it was actively promoted in Scotland and Northern Ireland but not in England and Wales. This meant that GPs in England and Wales were not made aware of it as a product available for use, and only doctors who had an interest in migraine knew about it. Eletriptan is listed in the *British National Formulary*, a book (revised every six months) that is used by health-care professionals, so your GP can look it up and check the doses suggested.

> **I want to try to find something that will stop my migraines happening at all. Can my GP help me with that?**

Your GP can help by explaining what drugs are available. A preventative drug will reduce the total number of attacks or headache days that you have but will not stop them completely. All drugs have the potential to produce side effects; whatever choice you make will be a trade-off between how effective the drug is and the side effects. Some drugs work better than others, and some people respond well to some drugs and not others. So you will probably have to try different options before finding the right one for you.

THE PRACTICE NURSE

My GP has said that I can contact the practice nurse for advice. How can she help me with my headaches?

The practice nurse will be able to offer you advice and support through the diet and lifestyle changes that you need to consider. Change is always difficult and support can be hard to find. Nurses are skilled in supporting patients through this process, and raising your headache and migraine threshold is crucial in getting back in control.

Some practice nurses have more knowledge about headaches than others. If they do have some experience with headache problems, they will be able to clarify some or all of the information given by your GP. The role of a practice nurse rather than a specialist nurse is of a more general nature.

I have been given a triptan by the GP for my migraine and he has suggested I see the practice nurse for review. What will the nurse do or want to know?

The nurse will want to know how well your treatment has worked, in order to be certain that you have found the best treatment for you. She will want to assess how the treatment has worked so that, if necessary, she can help you think about what else you might try.

The sorts of questions she will need to ask include:

- Did the triptan work quickly?

- Were there any side effects?

- If there were side effects, were they tolerable?
- Did the headache go away and stay away?
- Could you have taken your triptan any quicker?
- Would you like to try using a nasal spray instead of a tablet?
- Would you like to try a different triptan?
- Should you try something such as ibuprofen (anti-inflammatory and painkiller) or domperidone (to help with sickness) with your triptan?

I'll be working with the practice nurse to get my migraines under control. Can she prescribe anything for my migraine?

The best treatment for migraine is a triptan. The nurse will not be able to issue a prescription for a triptan but will be well placed to make suggestions or recommendations to the GP.

The practice nurse has given me some diary cards to use but I don't see how they can help.

The main reason for using diary cards is to see just how many headache days you have, assess what symptoms you get with your headache, work out how long your headache lasts and see how effective your treatment is.

It may seem like a chore filling in diary cards but it is a useful way of seeing what is happening to your headache symptoms over time. It can offer useful information or guidance on what options might be appropriate from both an acute and a preventative perspective.

***My GP has given me some diary cards to use and told me to
see the nurse for review. What will happen during that review
session?***

The nurse will use the time to determine how many headache days
you have had in each month, and see how well your treatment
works. Recording the time of the attack as well as the range of symptoms you experience will help plan new treatment options and
combinations of treatment. The aim is to be headache-free at two
hours with no recurrence of symptoms in the next 24 hours.

The nurse will use your diary cards to monitor how many
headache days you have and to see how these change over time if you
are using preventative treatment. The goal is to try to reduce the total
number of headache days by at least 50%.

***My practice nurse has given me some diary cards to use but
there does not seem to be much space to record what I eat and
drink. Is it worth making my own cards as well?***

There are lots of different sorts of diary cards available. Diary cards
can be a useful tool but I am always reluctant to use them as food
diaries. Headache is one of those situations with just too many variables to be able to offer you useful or even useable information. I feel
that it is more helpful to focus on positive steps such as having regular meals and drinking lots of water rather than documenting
everything you eat and drink.

For more information on food triggers, see Chapter 7.

***Having seen my GP, I'm now to see the practice nurse for
'review'. How often should I aim to see the nurse?***

There are two aspects to the review process. The first is about seeing how effective your acute treatment is, and the second is to
assess your response to preventative treatment.

Acute treatments are assessed after three attacks have been treated.

If the response is slow, incomplete or associated with too many side effects, alternative drugs or drug combinations can be suggested and then reviewed in due course. You will continue to go for review until you have found an acute treatment that suits you. The aim is to be headache-free in two hours, with no recurrence of symptoms within the next 24 hours.

Preventative drugs are usually assessed every three months. The number of headache days you have had is counted, and a dose increase suggested if your response is deemed unsatisfactory and few or no side effects have been experienced. You will keep filling in your diary cards until there has been an improvement in the number of headache days you experience or you have reached the maximum dose of the drug or the side effects you experience prevent a further dose increase.

> **I am seeing the practice nurse for her to check on how I'm getting on with the treatment. Will she eventually send me back to the GP?**

The nurse will send you back to the GP if and when she has run out of options to try. If you find an effective acute treatment, the GP does not need to see you. If you find a preventative drug that dramatically reduces the number of migraine attacks you have, you will only need to see the GP when it is time to stop taking them.

THE HEALTH VISITOR

> **Health visitors just deal with mums and young kids so how can she help my migraines?**

Health visitors do indeed provide support to mothers with young children. During this time in your life your migraine threshold will tend to be low and you will be vulnerable to migraine attacks. Your health visitor will be well placed to encourage you to think about potential triggers and to suggest changes and support strategies to help raise your threshold again.

My health visitor has been great helping me cope with my new baby. Do you think she could give me advice about my headaches?

Your health visitor is there to offer advice and provide support. She may suggest that you chat to your local pharmacist, see your practice nurse or visit your GP. She is there to guide you in the right direction so that you can find the right solutions. Having a new baby is hard work and full of new stresses and experiences. If you need help, do ask for it – trying too hard on your own may increase the number of headaches you get.

If you want to understand more about what sort of headache you have, see Chapters 2, 3 and 4. For advice on how to raise your migraine threshold, look at Chapter 7.

THE COMMUNITY MIDWIFE

One of the other mothers-to-be in my antenatal class has suggested that I ask the midwife for help with my migraines. What sort of help can a midwife offer me?

Your midwife is there to monitor your pregnancy and respond to anything that happens that could affect you or your unborn child. Migraine with aura may occur for the first time in pregnancy, and your midwife may suggest that you go to see your GP or recommend referral to a specialist if new or worrying symptoms develop.

If you want to know more about possible 'sinister' symptoms, look at Chapter 5.

Will the midwife be able to recommend a treatment for my migraine that is safe to use in pregnancy?

Your midwife will be aware of what you can take safely during pregnancy. She will also be able to discuss with you the relative risks involved in taking drugs during pregnancy and balancing these against the risks of not treating certain conditions or symptoms during pregnancy. It is a balance between pros and cons, of risk and benefit, and being active and well.

See also the section on pregnancy in Chapter 15.

What will the midwife do if nothing works for my migraine?

Your midwife will suggest that you go to see your GP if you continue to have problems with migraine while you are pregnant. Your GP may opt to refer you to a specialist if none of the acute treatments works or if you continue to have lots of headache days and need to think about prevention.

For more information on migraine and pregnancy, see Chapter 15.

WHO CAN OFFER SPECIALIST ADVICE?

A new GP at my health centre is listed as a GPwSI. What on earth is that?

A General Practitioner with Special Interest, or GPwSI, is a GP who has developed an interest and expertise in a particular area or speciality. For example, asthma or diabetes or heart problems . . . or headaches.

The GPwSI at my health centre is supposed to have a special interest in headaches. How could he help me?

As a GPwSI who specialises in headaches, he can make a full and detailed assessment of your symptoms, undertake an examination and decide what type of headache you have. It may be that your headache does not fit neatly in to a single diagnostic 'box' but fits partly into one of several boxes. If the diagnosis is straightforward, he will suggest a suitable treatment and management strategy. He will arrange to review you as appropriate.

If the diagnosis is less clear-cut or more complex, the GPwSI may refer you for investigation or send you to a neurologist for further assessment.

My GP says that he needs to refer me to a neurologist. What is a neurologist?

A neurologist is a doctor who has undergone formal training in neurology – diseases of the nervous system. The consultant will lead a team of doctors with varying levels of experience, all training to become neurologists. They are generally based within secondary care – usually a hospital. Some neurologists have a wide range of interests and are generalists; others develop a sub-speciality interest, such as headache, multiple sclerosis or Parkinson's disease.

My doctor wants to refer me to a neurologist at our local hospital. Why should I see a neurologist?

Your GP is just that, a generalist, not a specialist. A GP will be able to recognise and diagnose most common headaches. If your GP is not sure what is causing your headache or feels that there are some symptoms that don't fit into the diagnostic 'box', he will want you to be seen by a specialist. A neurologist will be able to exclude any serious or 'sinister' causes for your headaches, and will be best placed to support you if it is found that your headache symptoms are caused by some neurological condition.

If you want to know more about possible 'sinister' symptoms, look at Chapter 5.

Several of my friends get migraines, too. One of them is seeing a GPwSI and the other has been referred to a neurologist. Is a GPwSI better than a neurologist?

They both have a range of skills and expertise essential in managing and supporting the headache patient. A GPwSI with an interest in headache may be better placed to support a headache patient than a neurologist who is a generalist. A neurologist with an interest in headache is well placed to support headache patients with more a complex headache profile.

My GP has told me to liaise with the specialist nurse about my headaches. What sort of nurse would that be?

A specialist nurse is a nurse who has detailed skills, knowledge and expertise in a specific disease area. A nurse who specialises in headache is well placed to support the GPwSI, neurologist and patient from the point of diagnosis to discharge. Specialist nurses have a role in supporting people through complex decisions with regard to treatment and changes in diet and lifestyle.

How can a specialist headache nurse help me?

The specialist headache nurse will be able to support you when making choices about acute and preventative treatments. The nurse is also able to support you when stopping painkillers with a medication overuse headache – always a difficult and challenging time. She will encourage you to make changes in both diet and lifestyle to help your headache symptoms and support you while you are making those changes.

For more advice on tackling medication overuse headache, see Chapter 13.

The neurologist at the hospital has said he is going to refer me to a specialist, but I thought he was a specialist. Where is he going to send me?

A neurologist is a specialist in diseases of the nervous system but headache problems can be difficult and complex. There are super-specialist centres, or tertiary centres, where the more complex and rare disorders – in your case, headaches – are diagnosed and managed.

Where can I find out about what specialist centres there are?

The best sources are probably the Migraine Trust and the Migraine Action Association. They both have websites and patient support lines where you can seek out services that are available both nationally and locally. (Their contact details are given in Appendix 1.)

10 | What do the doctor and specialist nurse need to know and why?

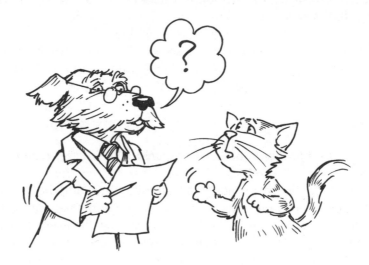

The first step in tackling your headache is making the diagnosis. The challenge is in trying to make the symptoms 'fit the boxes' as closely as possible – and, if they don't fit, deciding which box comes closest.

You will notice that this chapter is different from all the others. The questions are ones that I ask the patients I see rather than the questions that you might want to ask me. Every patient I see is different, and trying to understand your headache is never easy. Taking the history is about listening to your story, understanding your experience and distilling your answers in the hope that your headache fits into one of the 'boxes' from a diagnostic perspective.

The answer lies in the detail. I can make the diagnosis only if I can collect all the information, and the questions that follow are about all that information. Each and every question is a piece of the jigsaw and each piece has to be as clear and accurate as I can make it before looking for the next piece, and all the pieces have to fit together before a clear and accurate picture can be created. There are times when the edges blur and the pieces don't quite fit, in which case the boxes overlap just a little and they can't be completely separated.

Part of the assessment includes knowing something about you, your family and how you live your life. It is also important to know about what treatments you have tried before, what did and did not work as well as what you are using now and how effective it is.

If you want to get the most out of any consultation about your headache, or if you feel that the person you are seeing just doesn't seem to be asking the right questions, this chapter will help you get across all the detail needed to establish the right diagnosis.

WHAT THE DOCTOR NEEDS TO KNOW AND WHY

How old are you now?

Age is important because certain headaches are associated with particular times of life. People at different ages can have an increased risk of developing medical conditions that may give rise to headache symptoms.

How old were you the very first time you got a headache?

When you had your first-ever headache is important for a variety of reasons. A new headache that occurs for the first time later in life may indicate a serious problem – a 'red flag' – but if the headache occurred regularly in your teens or twenties and recurs later in life it is less likely to be serious unless the symptom 'profile' has changed dramatically. (For more information on 'red flags', see Chapter 5.)

A high-impact headache that occurs for the first time in someone over the age of 50 could well be serious. For example, temporal arteritis is a potentially serious headache that tends to occur in later years and is less likely to happen in younger people.

Have the headaches been the same since they first started?

Headaches that follow a similar pattern over time are less likely to have serious implications than ones that rapidly develop new and dramatic symptoms. A rapidly worsening picture over days and weeks has greater potential for having a serious cause than one than that evolves over months and years. Symptoms that always occur on the same side may be more likely to be associated with a potentially serious cause than symptoms that occur on either side. (For more information on 'red flag' symptoms, see Chapter 5.)

If the headaches have changed, when did that change happen?

A change in headache symptoms can occur for a variety of reasons, and the timing of that change can be helpful in identifying potential triggers. A change in symptoms or the symptom profile may indicate a potentially more serious cause, and this may need to be investigated.

Has the change been gradual or was there something that could have triggered it?

The symptoms of the migraine can develop and evolve over time. The detail is important in understanding why change occurs and in excluding a potentially serious underlying cause. Life events and having another medical condition (or conditions) may well contribute to a change in the headache profile. The development of symptoms during the headache phase may or may not be serious but needs to be assessed carefully.

If the headaches are different, is it:

a. Where you get the pain?

The site of the headache is an important factor in evaluating the possible diagnosis or trigger. Is it one-sided or are both sides affected? Is the pain in the same place or is it different every time? Does it spread or move, or stay in the same place all the time?

b. What the pain feels like?

Is the pain now throbbing whereas it was a pressure or tightness? Do you have an ache all the time that becomes throbbing every now and again? The description of the pain is one of the criteria used by the doctor to form a diagnosis.

c. How severe the pain is?

The severity of the pain is a criterion used to differentiate between headache types. Understanding the nature of the pain and how it has changed is important in clarifying the diagnosis and deciding which 'box' your headache fits into.

d. How long the headache lasts?

The duration of the headache is a feature vital in separating one type of headache from another. The shift from episodic to daily or near-daily headache is a difficult one to manage. The duration of the headache is a feature relevant in planning a treatment strategy.

e. How often you get the headache?

An increase in the frequency of headache symptoms may indicate the development of a medication overuse headache or a chronic tension-type headache. A reduction in the number of headache days may suggest an improvement in the headache.

The rate of change is important. An increase over days and weeks rather than months and years is more likely to be associated with a serious than a benign cause.

f. A change in your aura?

Aura symptoms tend to follow a typical pattern and are often described as being *stereotypical* – repeated each time. A change in the pattern of symptoms does occur but if these are significant or dramatic, a more serious cause should perhaps be ruled out. The question

I have to ask myself is: could this be a stroke or mini-stroke or just part of your migraine? I have to rule out the serious cause before assuming that it is due to the benign cause.

g. A change in the pattern or sequence of symptoms?

New symptoms need to be set in the context of pre-existing ones as well as expected or acceptable ones. There tends to be a natural evolution with migraine, visual symptoms being the most common aura symptoms, but sensory and speech changes can and do occur. Symptoms triggered by specific activities can be relevant, particularly if they are associated with a rise in intracranial pressure, such as results with coughing, intercourse or exercise.

Do you get any warning symptoms before the headache starts?

The warning phase may be the premonitory symptoms of mood swings, tiredness, yawning, irritability or food cravings, or an aura, which may have visual or sensory symptoms. Certain foods are often thought to be triggers but are more likely to be part of the premonitory phase in which food cravings form part of the start of the attack. The food craving leads to the food being eaten with the attack already on its way rather than the food causing the attack.

Knowing and understanding your premonitory symptoms or aura symptoms are useful predictors of the attack and allow you to treat it early.

Do you get an aura? If so, what do you see or feel?

An aura affects about in 1 in 10 people with migraine, and is most often visual but can be sensory. The symptoms of your aura are always completely reversible – they develop and go away without any active treatment. If you take the right treatment early enough, you might be able to shorten the length of your aura or even prevent your headache from starting.

Tell me what happens during your aura.

The aura is part of the migraine attack, and can vary from person to person. It may vary from attack to attack or change over time. The details are important, because a change in the symptom profile may indicate a potentially serious underlying cause that must be investigated.

It is helpful to make a note of the sequence of events and how long each set lasts, as this aids diagnosis.

- *a. Do you get your visual symptoms first? How long do they last?*

- *b. Do you get pins and needles or numbness next? How long do they last?*

- *c. Do they start with the visual symptoms or after? If after, how long after?*

- *d. Where do the sensory symptoms start? Hands, feet or face? Is your speech affected, now or later?*

- *e. What happens next?*

- *f. Do you get double vision? If you do, where do you see the second image? Is one eye or both eyes affected?*

What do you see during your aura?

Detail is important in assessing the nature of the aura and excluding retinal migraine from a more typical visual aura. The questions that follow allow that assessment to occur. Blurring of the vision is a premonitory symptom rather than an aura symptom.

- *a. Is it at the top, bottom, side?*

- *b. Does it move left to right, right to left, top to bottom, bottom to top?*

c. Is it black and white or coloured light?

d. Are both eyes affected or just one eye?

e. If you close your left/right eye, is the vision in the eye that is open normal?

How long does your aura last?

An aura should last no longer than 60 minutes and be completely reversible (i.e. it settles spontaneously and completely to normal). If it lasts longer than this, a potentially serious underlying cause may need to be excluded but a prolonged aura can be benign.

Does your headache start when the aura goes, or before?

In some people the headache may start before the aura settles, or the aura may not start until the headache does and can recur during the headache phase. Awareness of the sequence of events helps the doctor to determine the timing of acute treatment options. (See also the next question and explanation.)

Is there a gap between your aura finishing and your headache starting?

The headache of migraine may follow the aura immediately or within 60 minutes: this is migraine with aura. There are times when the aura is not followed by a headache at all, and is called aura without headache.

Does your headache start at a particular time of day or night? Or can it occur at any time?

The time of day that an attack starts can give clues to potential triggers such as falling blood sugar, hunger or dehydration. Posture and tiredness are also relevant.

Does your headache wake you up in the middle of the night?

Cluster headache tends to occur at night, as does hypnic headache, but being woken by the headache is a potential 'red flag'. This is one of the symptoms that need to be set in a context of time and previous symptoms. (For more information on 'red flags', see Chapter 5.)

Where do you get your headache?

The site or location of the headache is one of the features that form a 'diagnostic criterion', allowing one headache diagnosis to be separated from another. The questions that follow allow this to be evaluated in adequate detail.

a. Where does it start?

b. Does it move or spread?

c. Is it one-sided or on both sides?

d. Does it start on both sides and get worse on one side or the other?

What does the headache feel like?

Describing pain can be one of the hardest things for a headache sufferer to do but the doctor cannot diagnose the headache without knowing exactly what it feels like. Different headaches are associated with different types of pain and the following questions can help to clarify the headache character.

a. Sharp or dull?

b. Ache or pressure or tightness?

c. Squeezing or stabbing?

d. Throbbing, pulsating or pounding?

e. Burning or searing?

How bad is the pain?

The severity of the pain is a useful guide to what the headache might be. Mild or mild to moderate headache tends to be of relatively low impact and is more likely to be a tension-type headache than migraine or cluster headache.

A moderate to severe or severe headache is more likely to be migraine or cluster headache than tension-type headache.

Separating severity from what the pain feels like is difficult but crucial in trying to decide which diagnosis to make, and therefore which treatments are likely to be best.

Is the pain constant or does it come in waves or build to a peak before subsiding?

Understanding what the pain does when present helps the doctor to understand the underlying cause and, potentially, the diagnosis.

How long does the pain last?

The duration of the headache is another of the factors used to make the diagnosis – short, sharp neuralgic pain, as opposed to episodic migraine headache, compared with more chronic headaches. The following questions aid the process of determining the type of headache.

a. Seconds?

b. Minutes?

c. Hours?

d. Days?

e. Several days?

f. Several weeks?

Once the headache has gone, are you back to normal straight away, or does it take you a while to recover?

A slow recovery adds to the impact of the attack by prolonging the process. Understanding the impact and duration of symptoms aids decision-making for both acute and preventative treatments and for evaluating how effective they are.

How often do you get the headache?

It is important to understand the frequency and periodicity (or pattern) of headache symptoms. Is it a neuralgia, or a cluster or a tension-type headache? Is this an episodic or a chronic headache? Knowing the time of day or the day in the week the headache occurs may help in determining the triggers and therefore suggesting management approaches. The following questions aid the assessment process.

   a. Does it happen at some part or time of every day?

   b. Does it happen all day every day?

   c. Does it happen once every week, month or year?

   d. Does it seem to happen seasonally?

   e. Does it happen around the time of your period?

   f. Does it seem to be on a particular day of the week?

   g. Is it always at weekends or the start of a holiday?

How many headache days do you get each week, month or year?

This is one of those fail-safe questions to help determine the frequency issue. The frequency of the headache and the frequency with which an acute treatment is used are important in separating a chronic episodic headache from a more chronic daily headache from a medication overuse headache.

The follow-up question is 'Do you treat every headache you get?' A 'Yes' to that, on the back of a daily or near-daily headache, suggests the possibility of a medication overuse headache.

Does the headache make you feel nauseated or vomit (feel sick or be sick)?

Nausea and vomiting are symptoms typically associated with migraine, which is an episodic headache. If there is a daily or near-daily headache with occasional nausea, this could be a medication overuse headache with breakthrough migraine.

Nausea and vomiting early in the attack will affect how well your acute treatment works and which delivery system is best suited to treating the migraine. Understanding the subtlety of the blend and timing of these symptoms is essential in making the diagnosis and planning management.

a. Do you feel sick every time? Or not?

b. What percentage of episodes do you feel sick?

c. What percentage of episodes do you actually vomit?

d. How soon after the attack starts do you start to feel sick?

e. How soon after the attack starts do you start to vomit?

Are you sensitive to light, sound or smells during an attack?

Sensitivity to light, sound and smell are symptoms typically associated with migraine. The blend and balance of symptoms will vary according to the primary diagnosis and whether or not more than one sort of headache is being experienced.

a. Is this with all your headaches?

b. Or with some of your headaches?

c. Is it during your warning phase or aura?

Do you get any diarrhoea with your headache?

Diarrhoea is not a symptom that is often volunteered but is one that can be experienced. It is important to know about it, as it may affect the choice of medication tried for treating the attack: a suppository becomes somewhat futile and an injection or nasal spray more effective.

Do you feel hungry or lose your appetite with your headache?

Loss of appetite tends to be associated with migraine. Hunger may suggest that the attack is waning and recovery is on its way.

Does anything make your headache worse?

Migraine sufferers choose to keep still, cluster headache sufferers have to pace around. If you have neck or back problems, certain actions or activities may increase muscle spasm and lead to headache symptoms.

a. Coughing, sneezing, bending or exercise?

b. Specific activities or movements – e.g. painting, gardening, ironing, making the bed?

Has anything brought the headache on like a bolt from the blue, like a sledgehammer, and stopped you dead in your tracks?

Movement may well make a headache worse but causing or triggering the headache is a potential 'red flag'. Is a headache triggered during exercise related to low blood sugar or dehydration or something more serious? Teasing out these symptoms and what they mean requires patience and perseverance.

a. Coughing, sneezing or bending?

b. Intercourse?

   (i) If during intercourse, is it before, during or after orgasm?

   (ii) Is the headache the same or different from your usual one?

(iii) How long does this headache last?

(iv) Do you need to treat it or does it settle on its own?

c. Exercise?

(i) Is it any type of exercise?

(ii) Is it every time you exercise?

(iii) Do you have to exercise at a particular intensity?

(iv) Is it always after you have been exercising for a particular length of time?

(v) Is the headache the same or different from your usual headache?

(vi) How long does this headache last?

(vii) Do you need to treat it or does it settle on its own?

Have you ever been paralysed with the headache? Not in the sense of not wanting to move but being physically unable to move.

Paralysis is one thing, and a feeling of heaviness or weakness is another. Paralysis may be due to hemiplegic migraine, a transient ischaemic attack (TIA, a mini-stroke) or a stroke. Progressive symptoms of paralysis may indicate a structural lesion within the brain. Symptoms always occurring on the same side, even if reversible, may be signs of a structural lesion in the brain.

Detailed questioning is the only way to tease out the symptoms and understand the underlying pathology or pathophysiology – the causes and effects of the processes associated with a given condition. The precise details or sequence of events offers clues as to which part of the nervous system may be involved in generating the symptoms being experienced.

a. If you have been paralysed:

(i) When did you first experience this symptom?

(ii) Was it your face, hand, arm, foot or leg?

(iii) Was it one side or both sides?

(iv) How long did the symptom last?

(v) Did it happen before the headache or with the headache?

(vi) How often has it happened?

(vii) If it has happened more than once, is it always the same side or does it vary from attack to attack?

(viii) What is the exact sequence of symptoms?

(ix) Does it happen with every headache or just some of them?

(x) Does the symptom settle before the headache does, with the headache or after the headache?

Do you have any pins and needles, tingling, numbness or other changes in sensation?

These 'sensory' symptoms can occur as part of the aura or start during the headache. The symptoms have to be completely reversible, spontaneously, during the course of the attack and should settle before the headache does. Sensory symptoms may occur as a result of other medical, neurological or orthopaedic conditions; for example, carpal tunnel syndrome or sciatica, or even a brain tumour if it is in the right part of the brain. Teasing out the details is crucial in ruling out a potentially serious or structural cause.

a. When did you first experience this symptom?

b. Exactly what symptoms do you have?

c. Do they affect your face, hand, arm, foot or leg?

d. Were they on one side or both sides?

  e. How long did the symptoms last:

   (i) seconds?

   (ii) minutes?

   (iii) hours?

  f. If it has happened more than once, is it always the same side or does it vary from attack to attack?

  g. What is the exact sequence of symptoms? How do they develop and evolve?

  h. How often do you get these symptoms?

  i. Do they happen before the headache or with the headache?

  j. Do they happen with every headache or just some of them?

  k. Do the symptoms settle before the headache does, with the headache or after the headache?

Is your speech affected?

Speech can be affected not only in migraine but also with a stroke or a transient ischaemic attack (TIA). Speech can be affected in the premonitory, the aura or the headache phase. Speech can be affected in a variety of ways, so the details need to be recognised, highlighted and understood.

  a. Does this happen during the aura or warning phase?

  b. Does it happen with the headache?

  c. Is it there all the time or does it come and go?

  d. How is your speech affected:

   (i) slurring?

   (ii) jumbling of your words?

   (iii) coming out with the wrong words?

Do you have any dizziness symptoms?

'Dizziness' is a very subjective word. To make an accurate diagnosis, the doctor needs an objective, descriptive view, so it is important to describe this symptom clearly. Dizziness is a symptom associated with diseases of the ear, nose and throat (ENT) as well as neurological disease.

a. What do you mean by dizzy:

   (i) spinning?

   (ii) unsteadiness?

   (iii) feeling drunk?

   (iv) feeling light-headed or 'spaced out'

b. Have you fallen?

c. Do you tend to fall or veer in a particular direction?

What effect does the headache have on you?

Its impact on you is one of the most important distinguishing features of headache symptoms. Migraine makes you stop, cluster headache makes you pace, and different headaches do different things.

a. Do you sit still?

b. Do you lie down?

c. Do you want a quiet place?

d. Do you need a quiet, dark place?

e. Can you carry on as normal?

f. Do you have to pace around?

g. Does moving make the headache worse or better?

Do you eat regularly?

Eating regularly is important and, in the presence of other unavoidable triggers, may be all it takes to keep your threshold up enough to prevent a migraine.

a. Do you have breakfast, lunch and dinner every day?

b. Do you have snacks between meals?

c. Do you have a snack before bedtime?

Are you a food junky or do you have a healthy diet?

The quality of what you eat can be as important as the frequency with which you eat. A healthy diet and a healthy lifestyle can combine to result in a higher migraine threshold, which means potentially fewer migraine attacks.

Do you avoid or exclude any particular foods?

A balanced diet is important to provide the essential food groups as well as vitamins and minerals needed for a healthy body. A healthy body usually means a healthy and happy person, which means fewer headaches and fewer migraines.

Excluding a wide range of foods and food groups tends to lead to a very narrow and restricted diet, lacking the full range of vitamins and minerals needed for a healthy body. A true food trigger is rare and usually self-evident. Food cravings during the premonitory phase do occur and can easily be mistaken for a trigger of the migraine rather than part of the attack process, which has already started when you get your craving.

For more information about your diet, see Chapter 7.

Do you drink plenty of fluids?

Dehydration can cause headache, as can too much caffeine. It is possible to get a rebound headache from caffeine withdrawal. Artificial sweeteners may contribute to headache symptoms, so what you drink is as important as how much.

a. How many cups of tea or coffee do you drink each day?

b. Do you have caffeinated or decaffeinated hot drinks?

c. Do you drink Coke or Pepsi?

    (i) caffeinated or decaffeinated?

    (ii) low cal or regular?

    (iii) how many cans or bottles each day?

d. Do you drink water?

    (i) flavoured or not?

    (ii) how many cups, glasses or bottles?

e. Do you drink any other drinks?

f. Do you drink alcohol?

    (i) do you drink wine, beer or spirits?

    (ii) how many units each day, week or month?

What hobbies or interests do you have?

Having a balance between work, chores and play is crucial to feeling well and being happy. A happy and contented person will tend to have a higher migraine threshold than one who is too busy and too stressed. Having some time that is devoted to being 'me' is important in being and feeling in control.

What things cause you worry, stress or anxiety?

Stress can be both positive and negative. Recognising the highs and lows means you can get the balance right and stay in control. Knowing when your limits are being stretched or over-stretched means knowing when to ask for help and actually doing it.

How do you manage your headache?

Headaches are all different, and how we deal with them varies. Knowing what works for you is important, as is finding new things to try that might work better.

What do you take to treat your headache?

There are a range of treatments available to manage the wide variety of headaches. Knowing what to take for what sort of headache is essential, as the wrong treatment can cause more problems than it solves. Treating the headache is not just about treating the pain, but is also about tackling all the other associated symptoms that can be just as disabling.

   a. Do you take a simple painkiller?

      (i) What do you take?

      (ii) How many do you take?

      (iii) How often do you take it?

   b. Do you take something for the nausea and vomiting?

      (i) What do you take?

      (ii) Is a single dose enough or do you have to repeat it?

   c. Do you take a triptan?

      (i) Which one do you take?

      (ii) What strength or dose do you take?

d. Do you use a mix of tablets?

e. Do you take a single dose or repeat your dose of medication?

  (i) How often do you have to repeat your dose of medication?

For more information on acute treatments for headache and migraine, see Chapter 11.

When do you take your treatment?

When you take your treatment can be as important as what you take. Timing is everything – too early can be as ineffective as too late.

a. Is it with the aura?

b. With the warning phase?

c. With the start of the headache?

d. After the headache has been present for an hour, a few hours or several hours?

How effective is your treatment?

Everyone has a different goal when it comes to measuring how effective their treatment is. How quickly something works is relative to how long the headache would have lasted without treatment. A sustained response varies as much with early treatment as what drug is used. Drugs used in combination may be a better solution than one on its own.

a. Does it stop the headache from developing?

b. Does it ease the headache?

c. How long does it take to ease the headache?

d. Does it get rid of the headache completely?

e. How long does it take to get rid of the headache?

f. Does the headache come back in the next 24 to 48 hours?

g. Does it get rid of any or all of the other symptoms?

h. Do you get any side effects?

i. If you do get side effects, how bad are they?

j. If your treatment is effective, can you put up with the side effects?

How many days in the week do you take an acute treatment?

This is another question designed to discover the person with medication overuse headache, as they are usually reluctant to admit to exactly how many tablets they take!

Do you take a single dose in the day or more than one?

It is important to know exactly how many doses are needed for effective treatment. The goal is a drug or drug combination that works quickly, relieves all of the symptoms, has few or no side effects, is easy to use and does not allow the headache to recur.

WHAT THE SPECIALIST HEADACHE NURSE NEEDS TO KNOW AND WHY

The specialist nurse is there to assist and support you in your understanding of your symptoms, diagnosis and treatment. Your nurse is there to provide you with the information you need to make your choices and decisions, to allow you to get back in control of your headache symptoms, no matter how long it takes.

There are currently only a few such nurses in the UK, so these questions could be asked by your GP or your practice nurse or even friends and family after you have seen the specialist.

Do you understand what the specialist has said to you?

The nurse wants to make sure that you do understand what the provisional diagnosis or options are. The nurse also wants to be sure that you understand the strategy that has been suggested or outlined. The nurse will want and need you to feel involved and engaged in the process in order to give you back control of your headache symptoms.

Do you understand the diagnosis?

The biggest hurdle in diagnosis is the concept of medication overuse headache. Many people find that the diagnosis of migraine, cluster headache and other similar headache types are much easier to come to terms with than the diagnosis of medication overuse headache.

Let's talk about your meal patterns.

The nurse needs to understand how you eat during the day in order to offer you advice on what could be changed. Small changes can make big differences.

What sort of drinks do you have?

What you drink is as important as how much you drink. The nurse will spend some time going through the detail before making suggestions that might help you to raise your migraine threshold.

What sort of changes are you ready to make?

The process will mostly be about change. Small changes can be as powerful as, and produce a larger improvement than, the big changes. The changes will be about what drugs you take, what foods you eat, what drinks you drink, what hobbies you pursue. The steps will be small and manageable. The nurse will want you to decide what changes you feel you can make, when you feel you will be ready to make them and how you plan to make them.

What are you taking for your headache now?

The nurse will want to know what you are currently taking and how effective it is before suggesting ways of improving the result. The more effective your treatment, the fewer doses you will need. The fewer doses you need, the less likely you are to develop a medication overuse headache.

These are the options that the specialist has suggested – what do you think?

The nurse will work through the suggestions and recommendations made by the specialist. The nurse will then discuss with you the option that you feel best meets your needs. The choice has to be yours, the decision must be yours: the nurse is there to act as a sounding board and to answer your queries to help you make that choice. (See also the next point.)

Which of these do you feel best suit you?

The nurse will explain to you the range of drug and drug combinations available to treat an attack. There will be variations between how quickly the drugs work, the side effects experienced and the sustained pain-free effect achieved, and you will have to decide which you think will best meet your needs. This decision may well be modified by what you have tried already and what effect they had.

The choices and decisions are yours to make; the nurse's role is to make you aware of what options are possible and how those options and combinations might work.

Do you want to take a preventative drug?

Not many people want to take a tablet every day without a guarantee that it will fix all their headaches. The nurse's role is to explain why using a preventative drug might be a good idea for you. The nurse will then discuss the drugs available and review the suggestions made by the specialist and talk you through them. The choices and decisions are, as always, yours to make.

The nurse will explain to you that you do not have to take a preventative drug forever. It is there to reduce the number of headache days you are getting at the moment. She is likely to monitor things in three-month time blocks and, once things are stable, think about stopping the drug after six, possibly twelve, months of regular use at an effective dose.

What do you expect from a preventative treatment?

You need to set realistic goals when it comes to considering treatment options. The nurse will explain that diet and lifestyle changes can dramatically reduce the total number of headache days you have. Once you have made these changes, you may need to consider preventative drugs to produce a further reduction. You will not become headache-free with preventative drugs, but you should have many fewer headache days.

Different drugs work differently in different people and may work better for some types of headaches than for others. The 'side effect profile' will vary from drug to drug as well as from person to person. Choices are not always easy but the effects can be quite dramatic.

Would you like to speak to me again in a few days or weeks?

The nurse has a crucial role in supporting you through the process. Making changes and sticking to them is never easy, as life is busy and gets complicated. There are times when the changes just don't seem to be working, or are going too slowly. Motivation can be hard to find and almost impossible to sustain, but the nurse can be there to give you the gentle nudge you need. These contacts are likely to be via the telephone rather than face to face.

When shall I see you again?

The nurse will arrange a face-to-face review at regular intervals that allow you to reflect on the options you have chosen. This may be at one, two or three months, sometimes longer depending on how things are going. You can decide when that should be.

These are the diary cards we would like you to keep.

Diary cards are a useful way of discovering patterns or potential triggers as well as assessing your response to treatment. Diary cards vary, and therefore acquire different pockets of information. Centres often create their own diary cards whilst others use standard cards already available.

You and the nurse need to decide exactly what information you are going to record and how accurately you plan to complete your diary. Diary cards are a tool to be used to support and assess the options you have chosen and to help in deciding what to try next.

The specialist has suggested that you have a medication overuse headache. Do you understand what that means?

The nurse will explain to you what medication overuse headache is and why you need to stop taking the painkillers you have been using. This is one of the hardest concepts to grasp and the nurse can support you during the 'washout', or withdrawal, phase.

You need to stop taking all the painkillers you are currently taking. Do you think you can do that?

Everyone feels differently when told that they have to stop the painkillers they are taking. A series of conscious and determined choices and decisions have to be made. The 'cushions' that are put in place to support the process are different for every single person the nurse sees. The nurse's skill is in helping you find the 'cushions' that you need to succeed.

a. What steps do you think you need to take to be successful?

b. How do you think you can do it?

For more information on tackling medication overuse headache, see Chapter 13.

Do you want to take a preventative drug to support you during the washout?

Painkillers are not the only way of managing pain symptoms. There are several drugs or classes of drugs that can be used during and after your washout phase to help control the pain of your headache and that will reduce the need for you to take painkillers and contribute to successfully completing the washout.

The nurse will discuss with you the range of drugs available and talk through the doses and side effects as well as the effectiveness of these drugs. You will then need to decide which, if any, you feel you want to try.

When do you want to speak to me or see me again?

Making change is never easy, and having support is crucial to success in getting back in control, whatever the cause of your headache. A telephone call when things are getting tough might make all the difference to getting through the crisis. The nurse can make the difference between completing the washout successfully and not getting there, between treating your headache effectively and not getting the best effect.

The nurse can answer your questions, reassure you about side effects and make suggestions about what to try next. The telephone can be as valuable as a face-to-face consultation. Time is often an issue and a telephone chat could be a quicker and easier option and just as effective, especially if diary cards can be faxed (or perhaps even emailed) through in advance of the telephone consultation.

11 | Acute treatment

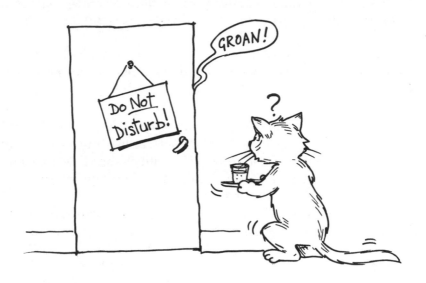

There are lots of different headaches and there are lots of different ways of treating those headaches. The important thing is to find the right treatment for the right headache. If you use the wrong treatment, it is not likely to work well and will lead to a sense of frustration, and can often make the headache worse rather than better.

Different treatments work differently for different people at different times. Finding the right treatment takes time, motivation and patience. Sometimes drugs can work best when taken alone, and sometimes they work best when used together with other drugs. There is no easy way of getting it right. If one treatment does not work, you could seek advice from your local pharmacist, ask your practice nurse or go back to your GP. The important thing is to keep trying. It may be that you will need to contact your specialist nurse, who may be able to offer advice or talk to the headache specialist.

ACUTE TREATMENTS FOR MIGRAINE

I've been taking ergotamine for years, as it's the only thing that really stops my migraine headache. I feel really dopey afterwards, though. Is there anything else I could try?

Ergotamine is a drug that is associated with a lot of side effects. It can be very effective but can build up in the system if you take it too often. There are lots of other options. Choosing the right one is not always easy and rather depends on what you have tried before.

You need to find a drug that works quickly, makes the headache go away and stay away and causes few, if any, side effects. Any simple painkiller taken with an anti-nausea drug might help. If that isn't any good, a triptan might work better. (There is more information on different triptans later in this chapter.)

Talk to your doctor about the possibilities and which ones you could try out.

My friend says that Nurofen (ibuprofen) works well for her migraine, but I don't find it helps me. Why doesn't it work so well for me?

There are several possible reasons for this. First and foremost, any given drug can work differently in different people. It is impossible to predict how one person will respond to a particular drug. All you can do is see how you respond – which in your case with ibuprofen is not very effectively.

You might do better if you take the ibuprofen a little sooner in the attack or perhaps try a higher dose, starting at the usual 400 mg and sometimes going as high as 800 mg. It might be that you need something like metoclopramide or domperidone to help the stomach empty and so absorb the ibuprofen better, especially if you feel sick early in your migraine.

I feel sick within a few hours of my migraine starting and I vomit back any tablets I take. Is there anything I can do?

Tablets used for nausea and vomiting can work if you get them in quickly enough. Timing and speed are the crucial factors! If it takes a few hours for the nausea to kick in, the tablets should work OK. There are two drugs that are designed to help the stomach empty and so help any painkiller you take be absorbed: metoclopramide and domperidone.

If you feel nauseated within 30 minutes, you might want to think about a suppository, provided you don't get any diarrhoea. Domperidone comes as a suppository as well as a tablet and can work as quickly as an injection.

What's the difference between Paramax and MigraMax?

The 'max' bit in both is from a drug called metoclopramide (brand name Maxolon), which is used to prevent nausea and vomiting. The 'Para' bit of Paramax is paracetamol. The 'Migra' bit of Migra-Max is a form of aspirin, which dissolves easily in water and works well when added to metoclopramide.

Is Nurofen different from Nurofen Migraine or is it just the same?

There is a difference between Nurofen and Nurofen Migraine. It is a biochemical one that means that Nurofen Migraine is absorbed into the system more quickly, which is really important in treating migraine. The basic painkiller in both, though, is ibuprofen.

I always start yawning and feel really tired for a few hours before my migraine starts. Is there anything that I can take that might stop my headache starting?

The yawning and tiredness are part of your premonitory, or warning, phase at the start of your migraine. If you can take something such as aspirin or ibuprofen, at a high enough dose (with domperidone or metoclopramide), as soon as you become aware of your symptoms, you stand a fair chance of preventing the headache from starting. If the headache does start, it might be less severe and settle with a second dose of medication.

I find that Nurofen Migraine seems to work quite well but the headache always comes back. Is there anything I can do?

When treating migraine, the headache can come back in up to 30–50% of attacks. This is more likely to happen if you delay treatment for any reason. One of the things you could do is take the treatment as soon as possible after the attack starts, which may be in the aura or the premonitory phase or when the headache itself starts.

If you already do that, the alternative would be to repeat Nurofen Migraine after four to six hours, which could stop the headache coming back. Alternatively, you could take something such as domperidone or metoclopramide to improve the way the Nurofen is absorbed.

It may be that you need to try something different such as a different anti-inflammatory, ibuprofen being one of many, or a triptan, which is a different way of treating migraine.

How many Nurofen (ibuprofen) can I take to get rid of my migraine?

I can't tell you how many, as that rather depends on the strength of the tablet. In an adult the standard dose is 400 mg but you might do better with 600 mg or 800 mg as your initial dose. The tablets come as 200 mg or 400 mg if you buy them 'over the counter' (i.e. without a prescription) from your local pharmacist. Your GP can prescribe 600-mg-strength tablets. There are also 800-mg-strength tablets but these are slow release and not suitable for migraine treatment.

> *I don't get an aura so I can't anticipate or predict a migraine. My doctor prescribed an anti-inflammatory and dihydrocodeine for when the pain has already started. Is this the best thing to take? They seem very strong and really knock me out.*

Migraine is an inflammatory process, so the anti-inflammatory is a good idea. The stomach also stops working so you need to take a 'gastric-emptying anti-emetic' (anti-nausea) to help things along. The dihydrocodeine is a very strong painkiller but has no anti-inflammatory activity and can make you very sleepy. It is good for other causes of pain but not really for migraine on its own.

> *Can I take paracetamol as well as ibuprofen to treat my migraine?*

Yes, you can, if it helps you. There are times when both drugs taken together can work better than one or the other on its own. Migraine is a process associated with inflammation, so anti-inflammatory drugs such as ibuprofen should work better than paracetamol, which does not have an anti-inflammatory action.

> *My migraine always comes back, even when it goes completely with my treatment. Why is that?*

The recurrence of headache symptoms happens for a variety of reasons. Migraine is a complex process in which symptoms can persist for up to three days. If you treat it early enough, you are more likely to completely suppress the process than if you delay treatment.

Preventing the headache from coming back at any time in the next 36 hours is about taking an acute treatment that is absorbed quickly and stays around long enough to suppress the progress of the migraine.

My treatment seems to work well for my migraine but the headache always comes back the next day. What can I do to stop that?

You could make sure that you take your treatment early enough, repeat the dose regularly through the first 24 hours, try a different drug, or add in an anti-nausea drug if you don't already take one.

If you are using a triptan, you could try a different triptan or a higher dose of the triptan you are already taking, or try a different formulation or delivery option. You could try a nasal spray or wafer instead of a tablet, or an injection instead of a nasal spray.

How can I stop my headache from coming back? I have tried a variety of treatments but they just don't make it go away. I feel as if I have some of the symptoms for three days, even though the headache is not so bad.

This rather depends on what you have tried already. The best way is to take an anti-inflammatory such as ibuprofen with domperidone as soon as your aura or warning phase starts, if you have one, and follow it up with a triptan as soon as the headache starts. If you do not have an aura or warning phase, take all three as soon as the headache begins. The earlier you start the treatment, the quicker it works and the more likely you are to get a sustained pain-free response.

If this does not work, repeating the dose of ibuprofen every six to eight hours through the first 24 hours usually puts a stop to it.

I have been to a headache clinic and they have said that I should try several different painkillers until I find which one works. How can I decide which is best?

The best is what you want it to be. It may be the one that works quickest, that lasts the longest and keeps the headache away or gets rid of all the symptoms. It may be that you can cope with some side effects because the medication relieves enough of the symptoms to allow you to function at some level. If you try several different ones, you can make that decision for yourself.

I want a painkiller that works quickly for my migraine. Can you suggest any?

The speed with which the painkiller relieves your migraine depends on how quickly it is absorbed. The earlier you take your treatment, the quicker it will work. Using a soluble form will help it to be absorbed more quickly. If you take your painkiller with a drug that helps empty your stomach (domperidone or metoclopramide), the painkiller gets into the bloodstream more quickly so it can do its job more effectively.

Some patients tell me that they can't stand soluble tablets; they take an ordinary tablet with a fizzy drink and that works for them.

There is more information about triptans rather than painkillers later on in this chapter.

What's the best time to take my painkiller to make sure the migraine gets better?

The simple answer is: as early as you can. Always have your treatment with you, so that you can take it as soon as you feel your symptoms starting. The more you delay, the longer it takes to be absorbed and the less likely it is to completely relieve your symptoms.

My GP has said that an anti-inflammatory is better than paracetamol to treat migraine. Why is that?

Research has shown that inflammation is part of the changes that happen in the brain during a migraine attack. Logic and research suggest that an anti-inflammatory is more likely to help migraine in more of the people more of the time than a painkiller such as paracetamol.

Can I take more than one dose of painkiller for my migraine headache?

If you get a migraine every now and again and it works well, then yes, you can. If you get migraine every week, though, how many painkillers you take becomes an important factor. If you take too many painkillers that do not work well, there is a risk that you could develop a medication overuse headache.

Taking a multiple dose of acute treatment, if it reduces the total number of headache days, is good news provided you do not need to use them too often. 'Too often' is taking them on three or four days in a week.

How can I decide if my new treatment is better than my old one?

If you think it is better, then it is! In order to discriminate further you will need to ask yourself a series of questions:

- Does it work more quickly or have fewer side effects than the treatment you are taking currently?

- Is it easier to take than your current option?

- Does it do what you want it to do?

These are questions only you can answer. You are the best person to decide which treatment is better, which is how it should be.

The treatment I have been using for years does not seem to work as well any more. What can I do?

This is a difficult question to answer because there are potentially many variables that you need to think about. Below are some factors for you to think about and see if they apply to you. Discuss them with your GP, headache specialist or specialist headache nurse.

If you are using simple painkillers such as aspirin, paracetamol or ibuprofen (which is also an anti-inflammatory) to treat your migraine, they can become less effective as time passes. You may get a better effect using a different combination or even a different drug altogether.

If some of your attacks occur around the start of your menstrual period, you may need to consider a higher dose of the drug that you are using for these particular attacks to get the same effect as with attacks that occur at other times of your cycle. This will depend on which drug you are using.

If there are times when the pattern of your symptoms changes and you start to feel sick or vomit earlier in the attack, your treatment may well be less effective. You might need to add in something such as domperidone to ease those symptoms or to speed up absorption of your painkiller.

My treatment seems to work better for some attacks and not so well for others. Is there anything I can do to make it more consistent?

Getting the timing right is crucial when it comes to treating your migraine. Using the right drug or drug combination at the right time makes a real difference to its effectiveness.

You can help yourself by understanding the different phases of the migraine attack and then being able to recognise where you are during the attack so that you can time your treatment well.

Simple painkillers should be taken as early as possible in the premonitory or warning phase of the attack or aura. They can be taken later but will work better when taken as early as this. Some people find they work *only* when taken this early.

Triptans are designed to be taken when the headache itself starts, not during the premonitory or aura phases. They can work at any time during the headache phase but are most effective when taken as early as possible in that phase.

You will need to keep your treatment with you at all times so that you can use it as early as possible. You should then find that the response becomes more consistent.

I find that Migraleve works well for me but my GP has suggested I try a triptan. Why?

Migraleve is a compound painkiller that contains several active ingredients, including paracetamol, buclizine (for the nausea and vomiting) and codeine in the pink tablet to be taken as the attack starts, and just paracetamol and codeine, in the yellow tablet, if the medication needs to be repeated.

A triptan is a migraine-specific drug that has been developed to target receptors in the brain and brainstem that are involved in the migraine attack. Your GP probably feels that a triptan will be more effective than your current treatment in resolving your migraine. If you are not so sure, go back and talk to your GP about it so you fully understand why he has suggested that you change drugs. In the meantime, consider the following questions about how well Migraleve works for you.

- Are you headache-free after using Migraleve or does it just ease your headache?

- Are you headache-free within 2 hours of taking the Migraleve?

- Does the Migraleve relieve all of your symptoms?

- Does the attack come back in the next 24 to 48 hours?

If your answers indicate that the results could be better, it would certainly be worth trying a triptan.

My cousin has been put on something called a triptan for his migraines. What is it?

A triptan is a migraine-specific drug treatment. It works by targeting specific receptor sites in the brain and brainstem. It is designed to be taken as the headache starts and can relieve all the symptoms of the attack. It can have an effect when taken at any stage of the attack but is most effective when it is taken early.

The different types of triptans and the different doses and delivery systems (ways of taking them) are shown in Table 11.1.

Table 11.1 Triptans, their doses and delivery systems*

Triptan	Formulations and dosing
Almotriptan	12.5 mg tablet
Eletriptan	20 mg, 40 mg tablets Maximum single dose: 80 mg
Frovatriptan	2.5 mg tablet
Naratriptan	2.5 mg tablet
Rizatriptan	5 mg, 10 mg tablets 10 mg wafer
Sumatriptan	50 mg, 100 mg tablets 6 mg injection 20 mg nasal spray 10 mg adolescent nasal spray 50 mg, 100 mg RADIS tablet
Zolmitriptan	2.5 mg tablet 2.5 mg and 5 mg orodispersible tablet 5 mg nasal spray Maximum single dose: 5 mg

*Information from the *British National Formulary* (*BNF*), vol. 51, March 2006

My GP has given me a triptan for my migraine. How does it work?

Your triptan will attach itself to very specific serotonin (5-HT) receptor sites in the brain and brainstem (see Figure 11.1). By doing this it is able to counteract their effect and stop the migraine attack from developing further. This means that all the symptoms associated with your migraine go away.

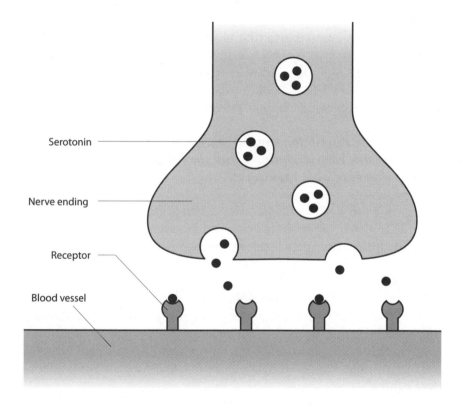

Figure 11.1 The 5-HT receptor sites on the vessel wall that release serotonin and are targeted by triptans.
(Adapted from *Target Migraine*, 2000, published by ABPI, London)

I'm using a triptan now and find it very good but our doctor won't let my son have any because he is only 16. Why is this?

Until recently, none of the triptans has been licensed for use under the age of 18. What do I mean by 'licensed'? Once all the research and trials have been done to assess how effective and safe a drug is, an application is made to the European Medicines Evaluation Agency for licensing. The licence specifies at what dose and for what conditions a particular drug can be used as well as what age groups it can be used in.

Recently, however, a particular formulation of sumatriptan as an adolescent nasal spray has been launched. This has been designed for use by 12- to 18-year olds. Another triptan called zolmitriptan is also available for use in 12- to 18-year olds. If you go back to your GP now, I am sure that she will be happy to discuss this with you.

I went to see my GP for some help with my migraines and he suggested I try a triptan. I read the list of side effects and I am concerned about taking it.

Triptans are a very effective way of treating migraine. The side effects listed may possibly occur but do not affect all of the people all of the time. Some people get no side effects at all, and others feel that the side effects they get are worth the benefit of an effectively treated attack.

The reason triptans cause this range of side effects is that they attach themselves to nerve receptors in all parts of the body, although they attach themselves best to the receptors within the brain. Different triptans can cause different side effects in different people, although studies suggest that some are less likely to cause side effects than others.

If you are concerned, go back and have a chat with your GP about it. It would be a shame to miss out on something that may cause you no problems whatsoever while getting rid of your migraine well.

The triptan I am taking gets rid of the headache of my migraine but makes me feel quite unwell. Is there anything I can do?

Any triptan can cause side effects in some of the people some of the time. But there are some that have been found to be less likely than others to cause problems. It is, however, impossible to predict how any one person is going to react. Almotriptan and naratriptan are associated with the least side effects, so, if you have not tried either of these, they might be worth a go.

You could also ask yourself whether, with the headache gone, you are perhaps just more aware of the other symptoms, rather than your symptoms being a side effect of the medication. I would encourage you to reflect on these options before giving up on the triptan.

What sorts of side effects should I expect to get when taking my triptan?

The side effects that you get are because the triptans target receptors on all blood vessels but have their maximum effect on the blood vessels in the brain. You may not get any side effects at all, but if you do experience problems the sorts of symptoms you might expect include:

- tingling or other sensory changes
- a feeling of heat
- a feeling of heaviness, pressure or tightness affecting any part of the body, most notably the throat or chest
- flushing
- dizziness
- a feeling of weakness or fatigue
- nausea and vomiting
- dry mouth
- indigestion or dyspepsia

If you do experience any of these side effects, have a chat with your GP. Each triptan is different and how you react to them will vary, so it is worth trying a different one to see if it suits you better, or try a lower dose if there is one.

I have just started using a triptan to treat my migraine. Are there any tablets or drugs that I should not take whilst using my triptan? It works really well and I just want to be prepared.

There are a variety of drug interactions that you should be aware of, and some of them are more likely to be an issue than others. Table 11.2 lists the drug interactions that are relevant.

Your GP is likely to be made aware of these when issuing the prescription, especially when using a computer as it routinely 'red flags' potential interactions. Your local pharmacist is also likely to be aware of possible drug interactions so if you have any concerns just check with them.

Table 11.2 Drug interactions with triptans*

Triptan	Drug interactions and precautions
Almotriptan	Ergot or methysergide: avoid for 24 hours after use Avoid St John's wort at the same time
Eletriptan	Avoid clarithromycin and erythromycin (antibiotics) Ergot or methysergide: avoid for 24 hours after use Itraconazole, ketoconazole (anti-fungal drugs): avoid concomitant use – risk of toxicity Indinavir, nelfinavir, ritonavir (anti-viral drugs): avoid concomitant use – risk of toxicity Avoid St John's wort at the same time
Frovatriptan	Fluvoxamine: may inhibit metabolism SSRIs: possible increased serotonergic effect Ergot or methysergide: avoid for 24 hours after use Avoid St John's wort at the same time

Table 11.2 Drug interactions with triptans* (*cont'd*)

Naratriptan	No significant drug interactions listed
Rizatriptan	MAOIs: avoid for 2 weeks after use of triptan Moclobemide (antidepressant): avoid for 2 weeks after use – risk of CNS toxicity Propranolol: use 5 mg dose Ergot or methysergide: avoid for 24 hours after use Avoid St John's wort at the same time
Sumatriptan	Increased risk of CNS toxicity with citalopram, escitalopram, fluoxetine, fluvoxamine (antidepressants) Sertraline: avoid concomitant use MAOIs: avoid for 2 weeks after use of triptan Moclobemide (antidepressant): avoid for 2 weeks after use – risk of CNS toxicity Ergot or methysergide: avoid for 24 hours after use Avoid St John's wort at the same time
Zolmitriptan	Quinolones (antibiotics): reduce dose of triptan MAOIs: increased risk of CNS toxicity Moclobemide (antidepressant): reduce dose of zolmitriptan Fluvoxamine (SSRI): reduce dose of zolmitriptan Ergot or methysergide: avoid for 24 hours after use Cimetidine: reduce dose of zolmitriptan Avoid St John's wort at the same time

*Information from the *BNF*, vol. 51, March 2006

I find that there are times when my triptan works better than others. Why is this?

Answering that question is not easy. Timing is the first thing I tend to check. If you take your triptan within one hour of the headache starting, it is likely to be more effective than if you take it later. Remember, too, that triptans are not designed to work if they are taken too early – during the warning or aura phase.

Triptans do not work for every attack, and they do not always work as well for some attacks as others. The reasons for this are not clear but probably reflect differences in the absorption of the drug during the early phases of the attack and also the variation that occurs from attack to attack in the normal course of events.

> *I went to see a specialist and he says I should take ibuprofen and my triptan together. I don't like taking too many tablets, though, so is this all right?*

If your triptan on its own isn't enough to completely stop your migraine, taking ibuprofen at the same time is a good idea. The two may well work better together than one or the other on its own. The idea behind using both is to reduce the total number of headache days you experience.

> *I always know when my attack is going to start but my triptan does not seem to work. Why is that?*

You may well know exactly when your attack is going to start, but if you take the triptan before the headache starts it is not going to work. You need to wait until the headache itself begins to get the best result from your triptan. Ideally, it should be taken within one hour of the headache starting.

> *Some of my attacks start with an aura and others do not. My GP told me to take my triptan as soon as my attack starts. I have found that this only works in the attacks that do not have an aura. I think I should wait until the headache starts. Am I right to delay treatment in that way?*

Yes, you are. Triptans work on very specific receptors and have been designed to work in the headache phase. Your GP is right, provided your attack starts with a headache and not an aura.

My GP has suggested that I try a nasal spray instead of my usual tablets. Why?

The most likely reason is to offer you a treatment that will work more quickly than the one you are currently using. A significant number of people have found that nasal sprays start to work within 20 to 30 minutes of being taken, so a spray is likely to work more quickly than your tablet.

My triptan always gets rid of my migraine headache within two to three hours but I find that it will usually come back later that day or sometimes the next day. Is there anything I can do to stop this?

Headache recurrence happens with a lot of migraine attacks. It occurs in part as a result of how the triptan works or the nature of the migraine attack itself; a migraine attack can last up to 72 hours. There are a variety of things that you might want to try.

First, check that you took your triptan as early as you could at the start of the headache. Secondly, if you get an aura or other warning symptoms, try something such as ibuprofen as soon as those symptoms begin. Another option is to take ibuprofen regularly through the rest of the day.

Is it better to take sumatriptan 50 mg or sumatriptan 100 mg?

When sumatriptan was initially developed it was launched as a 100 mg dose. This dose is very effective but can cause side effects (discussed a little earlier) and it has since been found that 50 mg can work just as well in some people. In the USA they use a 25 mg dose as well.

The best dose is the one that takes away your headache quickly, causes few or no side effects and does not allow the headache to come back within the next 24 to 48 hours. Only you can decide which one is better – not always an easy choice. You need to be confident that what you take will work well for you, relieving all of the symptoms of your attack and not allowing the symptoms to recur.

> *My specialist suggested that a nasal spray would be better for my migraine but I hate the taste that I get down the back of my throat. It seems to work really well, though, so is there anything I can do to help get rid of the taste?*

If you lean forward while you take the nasal spray rather than sit upright, it is less likely to trickle down the back of your throat.

You don't say which nasal spray you are taking. There are two different ones, so you could try the other one. If you don't get the taste problem but it doesn't work as well, then you'll have to decide what you want to do. Do you accept the taste with the one that works better or use the one that isn't quite as good but doesn't cause any problems? Only you can decide that one.

Have you tried a drink or sucking on a sweet afterwards? I know if you are feeling nauseated that might not be a good idea but it could be worth giving it a go.

> *I have tried three or four different triptans but none of them seems to work. Why is that?*

It depends on what you mean by 'not working'. If you mean it only eases the headache rather than taking it away completely, that may well be par for the course for the triptans you have tried. If 'not working' means no effect on your symptoms at all, again that simply reflects your response to those particular drugs. Are you perhaps taking it too early or too late?

Every single person has a different response to each of the seven triptans that are currently available. Each triptan works best if taken early in the headache phase or if taken with a painkiller/anti-inflammatory such as ibuprofen. The only way to find out which triptan suits you best is to try each of them for three consecutive attacks and then decide. You will need to enlist the help of your GP in prescribing them, but trying each triptan in turn is the only way you will find out.

My triptan gets rid of the headache but I still feel nauseated and very, very tired. Should I try something different?

Headache is only part of a migraine attack. The other symptoms are nausea, vomiting, and sensitivity to light and sound as well as poor concentration and tiredness. A triptan can treat all the symptoms of a migraine attack but there are times when the best it can do is relieve the headache.

The nausea can be treated by taking something such as domperidone or metoclopramide. These can be taken either before or at the same time as your triptan. The tiredness is slightly more problematic. Having a lie down in the first few hours of the attack may be the only option.

Even after the pain is gone, it takes another day or so for me to get better. Is this normal?

Yes, it is. It's called the recovery phase and can last several hours or the rest of the day. Some people feel tired, washed out and lethargic whilst others actually feel full of energy and the need to do things.

ACUTE TREATMENTS FOR CLUSTER HEADACHE AND PAROXYSMAL HEMICRANIA

Cluster headache is very different from migraine but, despite this, can respond well to triptans. The challenge with cluster headache is that each episode of pain can be very short-lived – so short-lived that no drug can work quickly enough to reduce the time the pain lasts. Only if the pain lasts for at least 30 minutes is it feasible to try a triptan, usually as a nasal spray or injection, to stop the pain once it has started.

I have tried lots of different painkillers to treat my cluster headache but none of them seems to work very well. Why is this?

Ordinary painkillers do not usually work well for cluster headache pain, mainly because they do not work quickly enough. An injection of something such as diclofenac may ease the pain, as it can start to work within 15 to 20 minutes of being used. Diclofenac suppositories can work almost as quickly if you can't face the thought of using an injection. The advantage of the suppository is that you can administer it yourself, rather than needing a doctor or nurse to give you an injection.

My GP has given me sumatriptan tablets but they don't seem to help very much. Why is that?

That depends on what you mean by 'very much'. Does it just ease the symptoms or does it have no effect at all? It may be that you need to increase the dose, from 50 mg to 100 mg, or you should swap to the injection or nasal spray, which will work more quickly and therefore help 'a bit more'. Your GP will not know it's not helping unless you go back to tell him. There are other options, so do go back to find out about them.

My cluster headache lasts up to an hour. What's the best thing to take for it?

The best would be the one that works quickly with the minimum of side effects. The quickest is likely to be an injection or nasal spray, but these may cause you unacceptable side effects. A tablet or wafer may cause fewer side effects but not work quite as quickly. Only you can decide which is the best.

My cluster headache usually lasts two to three hours.
My GP has given me sumatriptan tablets; do you think they
will work?

They should work if you take them quickly enough, and 100 mg is likely to work better than 50 mg. It may be that they will only ease the headache rather than take it away completely.

My cluster headache only lasts 10 to 15 minutes.
Is there anything I can take to help?

This is difficult because most treatments take this long to work. For cluster headache this short, oxygen tends to be the only option that has a chance of working quickly enough. Because acute treatment options are limited for such a short acute episode, you probably want to think about taking some preventative treatment (see Chapter 12). If you have episodic cluster, a short course of oral steroids is probably the best option for you, provided there are no reasons why you can't take them.

My specialist has suggested that I try oxygen to treat my
cluster headache. How do I go about getting a supply?

The very first time you need oxygen, a Home Oxygen Order Form (HOOF) has to be completed. This can be done by your GP or your specialist. The form is then sent to the contractor for your area or region, who will deliver the oxygen to your door. Your GP or specialist will also need you to sign a consent form so that your information can be held on file by the contractor supplying your oxygen.

At the time of writing, the contractors are:

- *Air Products* supplies North West, Yorkshire and Humberside, Leicestershire, Northamptonshire and Rutland, Trent, Birmingham and Black Country, Shropshire and Staffordshire, West Midlands, Wales, NE London, NW & Central London,

SW Peninsula, Dorset and Somerset, Avon, Gloucestershire and Wiltshire

- *Allied Respiratory* supplies SW & SE London, Thames Valley, Hampshire and Isle of Wight

- *British Oxygen* supplies Kent and Medway, Surrey and Sussex, Bedfordshire and Hertfordshire, Essex, Norfolk, Suffolk and Cambridge

- *Linde Gas UK* supplies County Durham, Northumberland, Tyne & Wear and Tees Valley

If I use oxygen, do I need a special regulator and mask?

You don't need a special regulator, because the high-flow valve is an integral part of the oxygen cylinder and is supplied with it. To treat cluster headache effectively you need a flow rate of at least 9 litres per minute of 100% oxygen, and this information must be specified on the HOOF in the 'short burst oxygen' part of the form.

The mask is special because you need one that has no holes in it. It will be supplied with your oxygen cylinder, provided it is listed on the HOOF.

My GP has just faxed my HOOF to our local contractor. I am in the middle of my cluster episode – how quickly can I expect the oxygen to be delivered?

The contractors supplying oxygen provide a 24-hour service, seven days a week. A routine supply will be delivered within three working days. In an emergency, your cylinder can be delivered within four hours.

I have been using oxygen for the last few years for my cluster headache. I have always got my oxygen from my local pharmacist. I know the regulations have changed. How do I get more oxygen when I need it?

Once your local contractor has received a Home Oxygen Order Form (HOOF) all you need to do is phone them direct, and they will arrange delivery. The contractor does not need to have a HOOF every time you need more oxygen.

My GP was trying to fill in my HOOF form and wanted to know how much oxygen I needed. How can I work it out?

In the past your GP would simply stipulate on your prescription a certain number of cylinders. On the new form the number of hours per day is what is needed. You need to base your calculation on your worst day. The total number of attacks and how long you use your oxygen will give you the number of minutes or hours that you use the oxygen; the contractor will then decide how many cylinders to deliver to last you three days.

I use oxygen five or six times a day when my cluster headache is at its worst. How will I know when I need to reorder my oxygen?

When your first oxygen supply is delivered, the agent will be able to show you where on the cylinder you need to get to before ordering more.

I have been told by the specialist that my headache is something called paroxysmal hemicrania. What is the best way to treat it?

Paroxysmal hemicrania is a unique headache in that treating it is easy. It responds well to a drug called indometacin. To control the symptoms of this type of headache, indometacin needs to be taken three times a day to a total daily dose of 150 mg.

If you want to know more about paroxysmal hemicrania, look in Chapter 3.

ACUTE TREATMENTS FOR TENSION-TYPE HEADACHE

Tension-type headache is very common, usually short-lived and best *not* treated with painkillers. If you do take painkillers to treat it, you should not run into any problems provided you get a headache only every now and again. However, the more headache days you have, the greater the chance you have of developing a medication overuse headache: if you always take painkillers for frequent tension-type headache, you will be taking them too many days in the week and running the risk of developing a medication overuse headache. This is when you need to think about other ways of treating the headache, including preventative drugs.

If I can't take painkillers to treat my tension-type headache, what can I do?

There are a variety of ways that you can try to ease the headache. You could massage where you feel the pain, perhaps adding in lavender or something like that to relax the muscles and ease the headache. Local heat using a wheat bag or something similar can also ease the headache. Everyone relaxes in different ways; what you have to do is take the first step and make the time.

If you want to find out more about raising your headache threshold, look in Chapters 7 and 8.

How often can I take painkillers to treat my tension-type headache before I am using too many?

This is a difficult question to answer until a variety of facts are considered! Too many depends on how many days you take your painkillers over time. Too many is not necessarily how many doses you take in a day but the number of days in the week that you take them.

If you take three doses in a day one day in the week, there is not likely to be a problem. If you take three to four doses in the day on two days in the week, again it is not likely to be too many. The 'too many' kicks in if you take one or two doses on four or more days in successive weeks. The shift from occasional headache to daily or near-daily is more likely to happen the longer you continue to use the painkillers with this regularity. What you don't want is your tension-type headache to become a medication overuse headache.

If I need a painkiller for my tension-type headache, which is the best one to use?

A simple painkiller such as aspirin, paracetamol or ibuprofen is better than a combination painkiller such as aspirin or paracetamol mixed with codeine or caffeine or both. The more potent the mix of drugs, the fewer days needed to hit the threshold for medication overdose headache to develop. The best advice is never treat low-impact headache with painkillers unless absolutely necessary. Try to ease your headache by using one of the many ways of 'relaxing' if you can.

12 | Preventative treatment

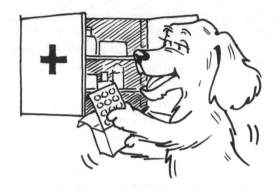

There are lots of different headaches and there are lots of different ways of treating them. The important thing is to find the right treatment for the right headache. This is true of preventative treatments as much as it is true of acute treatments. Choosing when to use preventative drug treatment will vary from person to person, and deciding which drug can depend on a host of different factors.

Remember that you don't have to take any preventative drug for ever, just for long enough to break the cycle of frequent headache days. This can vary and may be for as little as three months or as long as six to twelve months; only you can decide what works for you. You often have little to lose and much, potentially, to gain by trying preventative medication.

PREVENTATIVE DRUG TREATMENT FOR MIGRAINE

My GP has said that I need prophylaxis but I am not sure what it means. What is it?

P*rophylaxis* means 'prevention' and is used here to describe a drug taken on a daily basis to try to reduce the total number of headache days you are experiencing. In some people the attacks themselves can also become easier to treat.

If I take prophylaxis, will it stop all my migraines?

If you find the right drug and take it for long enough at the right dose, it can reduce the number of attacks you experience by at least 50%. It is unlikely to stop all of your attacks, though. The goal will be to reduce the total number of headache days you experience. You will still need an effective acute treatment for any breakthrough attacks that you may get. Remember: it will only stop some of the attacks some of the time.

Is preventative treatment any different from prophylaxis?

Preventative drug treatment and prophylaxis are just different words for the same thing. But preventing migraine is not just about taking tablets – it's also thinking about the other things that you can do to raise your migraine threshold so that you are less likely to trigger a migraine. These include looking at your diet and your lifestyle to see if any changes would help you.

If I opt for prophylaxis, do I have to take it every day?

Prophylaxis will work only if you take it at the prescribed dose every day. This may seem tedious but it is the only way to get the best effect from whichever drug you choose. You also need to be sure to take it for long enough and reach a high enough dose to have the desired effect.

How do I know what dose I need to take in order for a preventative drug to work?

You – and your doctor – won't know the right dose until you find it! Different drugs work differently in different people and at different doses. It is usually worth starting at the lowest dose, taking it for three months and then increasing the dose if you have not noticed any reduction in headache days.

'Start low and build slow' is a useful motto to follow to minimise side effects and allow you to find the right dose to reduce the number of headache days you have. If the first drug doesn't work, it is always worth trying a different drug in the same class, or try a different type of drug altogether.

If I take preventative drugs, how long do I have to take them?

You need to take them long enough to have an effect. This usually means taking a particular dose for three months before deciding whether that dose is making a difference. Having found a drug, and a dose, that does reduce the number of headache days you experience, it is not easy to decide the right time to stop them. Usually six months is enough to break the cycle and reduce the number of times an attack starts. (See also the next answer.)

If the headaches do recur, you could restart the medication or, if you have been slowly reducing the drugs, go back up to the dose that controlled your symptoms.

If prophylaxis works, how long can I take it for?

There is no benefit in taking it for ever. Six months is usually enough to break the cycle, once you have reached an effective dose. The reason for taking prophylaxis is to raise and then reset your migraine threshold. Deciding when to stop is about thinking where your threshold is and being aware of all the factors in your life that might push it down. If there are too many things around that push your threshold down, you might delay stopping your prophylaxis until things are a little more under control.

I have started on amitriptyline and been advised to increase the dose each week. Why so slowly – surely the quicker I get to the right dose the quicker I will notice an effect?

The main reason for increasing the dose slowly is to try to reduce the chance of side effects being a problem for you. It is one way of finding a dose that you can tolerate while reducing the number of headache days you have. Dose changes tend to be in small steps. The smallest step you can take with amitriptyline is 10 mg. The initial target dose is 30 mg daily; the next would be 50 mg. The maximum dose for amitriptyline is 150 mg in a day but this is rarely needed.

My friend has tried loads of different drugs but they all cause side effects with her. Is there any hope for me?

Everyone is different so there is no reason why you won't be able to find a preventative drug that works and does not cause unacceptable side effects. Any drug has the ability to produce side effects and the symptoms do vary from drug to drug. Most people are able to take a drug and experience no difficulties at all. Some people are more sensitive to drugs and become aware of side effects.

Side effects can vary according to the particular drug, the dose used, how often you take the drug and how quickly you build up the dose. Some side effects are more problematic than others and you will have to consider whether the benefits outweigh the disadvantages. Only you can decide but if you don't try you will never know!

My sister has found that every time she stops her preventative drug her migraines start again after three to four weeks. Why is this?

It is not really possible to say exactly why. Preventative drugs cannot stop migraines happening forever – a migraine can happen at any time. A preventative drug breaks the cycle when the number of migraines you get increases and they don't seem to want to settle down.

The frequency of your sister's migraines depends on a lot of factors, and thinking about where her migraine threshold is may provide the answer to why the migraines start up again with the same sort of frequency.

I have tried several different drugs to stop my migraines but none of them seems to work. Why is that?

There may be many different reasons why they don't seem to have worked. A major factor is that different people respond differently to drugs. You need to find the right dose of the right drug and you need to use it long enough for it to work. There are times when you need to do other things to push up your threshold so that the preventative drug gets a chance to work. Everyone is different and it may be that you haven't found the right drug yet or the right dose. So keep trying.

I have been given propranolol to help my migraine. The nurse at the clinic says I'll have to take it for three months before I'll be able to tell if it is helping. Why so long?

You might notice some improvement within the first week or two but some people take longer to respond. (Some people stop the drug too early because it doesn't seem to be working.) Taking the propranolol for three months at the lowest dose gives the drug a chance to have an effect at the lowest dose that will work. There is no point in taking a drug at too high a dose, as higher doses are more likely to cause side effects.

I have been talking to different people I've met at the clinic. One of them says that she took propranolol 80 mg and another said that he needed 240 mg. Why did it take such different doses to bring their migraines under control?

Essentially, everyone is different in how they respond to drugs. Propranolol works best if you have migraine and do not get any other headaches.

It is easier to remember to take a tablet every day if you only have to take it once a day. Propranolol can be taken just once a day because it is available as a slow-release preparation. The first dose routinely prescribed is 80 mg; this can be stepped up to 160 mg and then to 240 mg, and occasionally to 320 mg. Each dose is taken once a day for three months, and the dose is increased only if there has been no significant or acceptable reduction in headache days.

Every drug I have tried has resulted in my putting on weight. Are there any drugs that won't cause me to gain weight?

A lot of drugs can cause weight gain as a side effect, but not every- one necessarily experiences it as a problem. You have been quite unlucky to have had problems with all the drugs you've tried. The only drug used for migraine prevention that causes weight *loss* as a side effect is a drug newly licensed for use and it's called topiramate.

I have been looking on the internet and have read that there are beta-blockers other than propranolol to help migraine. Is it worth giving them a go?

Yes, it is. Beta-blockers are a group or 'class' of drugs that are usu- ally used to treat high blood pressure or ease anxiety symptoms as well as reduce the frequency of migraine attacks. They are all slightly different in how well they do this, although the effect they have is viewed as a 'class effect'. Some are seen as more likely to be of benefit than others on the basis of published research. Alternatives to propranolol include atenolol and metoprolol.

I have asthma so can't take beta-blockers, which worked for my mum. What else can I take?

Unfortunately, beta-blockers and asthma do not mix. If you want to try a preventative drug, you could try an anti-epilepsy drug or a tricyclic antidepressant.

If you want to avoid taking any preventative drugs, you might want to focus on diet and lifestyle changes. Have a look at Chapter 7 for different ways of doing this.

Why has my GP given me an epilepsy drug to stop my migraines?

Anti-epilepsy drugs (AEDs) are used to treat chronic pain and migraine as well as epilepsy. Crudely speaking, the anti-epilepsy drug is stabilising the brain and preventing it from causing the symptom. That symptom might be an epileptic fit, feeling pain or a migraine attack.

My GP said he was prescribing me Epilim but the box says sodium valproate; is it the same thing? It was Epilim that the specialist nurse suggested and I don't want to be given the wrong drug.

Epilim is the brand name of sodium valproate, so they are the same and you have the right drug. In general terms the 'names' are interchangeable. Most drugs these days are prescribed by their generic name but there are some exceptions when it is crucial to get exactly the right amount of drug in the bloodstream. and Epilim is one of them. Epilim is ideally to be taken twice a day as a slow-release preparation (Epilim Chrono). Using the brand name means that you know exactly how quickly, or slowly, the drug is released, so you know exactly how much drug is getting into the system, where it needs to be.

I was given a drug called Epilim that worked really well but my hair started falling out. My GP said that I would have to stop taking the drug but I am not keen as it has stopped my migraines. What are my options?

Hair loss is one of the side effects that Epilim (sodium valproate) can cause. Epilim is a drug used to treat epilepsy, and trying a different anti-epilepsy drug (AED) might give you the same benefit without this particular side effect. If you don't want to try a different AED, you might consider a beta-blocker or a tricyclic antidepressant. Of course, any of the alternatives can lead to side effects, but they will be different from those found with Epilim.

My sister put loads of weight on when she took Epilim. Will the same happen to me?

The simple answer to that is: not necessarily. One of the recognised side effects is weight gain but it doesn't happen to everybody. It is certainly worth trying but if you find that you do start to gain weight, stop it and try something different.

I am getting confused by all the different tablets my daughter has been given. She has been taking Epilim (sodium valproate) and some of the tablets are 200 mg and some are 300 mg, and they have 'Chrono' on the box. Why does she have different strength tablets? Or are they all the same?

'Chrono' is the bit of the name that tells you that it is a slow-release tablet. This means that you take the tablet twice a day. There are three Epilim Chrono tablets – 200 mg, 300 mg and 500 mg – so they are the same drug but they are different strengths.

I expect that your daughter was given the 200 mg tablets to start with, to see if she would get any side effects from the drug. It is usual to take this dose for three or four days before increasing it, perhaps to 300 mg as the next step. I usually do what I refer to as a 'slow up-titration' – increasing the dose in the smallest possible steps – to try to minimise any side effects that might be experienced.

My specialist nurse has told me that I need to have regular
blood tests when I start taking Epilim. Why is that?

Many drugs are processed by the liver, to break them down and inactivate them. In some people, the enzymes in their liver can be affected by these drugs and become overactive. In order to ensure that your liver is not being adversely affected, regular blood tests over the first few weeks and months is the only way to confirm this. If there is little or no change, it is safe to carry on taking the Epilim.

I have been taking Epilim for six months and have found
that my migraines got better initially, but they've become
more frequent again over the last few weeks. Is there a
maximum dose I can take?

The usual maximum dose for Epilim is 2g a day, usually in two separate doses. There is no right or wrong dose, and it is often worth going up to the maximum dose of 1g twice daily to see what works for you.

I have tried a couple of AEDs but they either did not work or
caused side effects that I found unpleasant. Are there any
other AEDs that work for migraine?

There are several different AEDs used for migraine prophylaxis. Epilim (sodium valproate) is one; others include topiramate, gabapentin and levetiracetam. Topiramate has recently been licensed for use in migraine prevention and is certainly worth trying. It may be that your GP will be happy to prescribe it, even though the current license advice is that it should be from a hospital specialist.

My friend has used topiramate for her migraine and it
worked really well. Could I try it?

Yes, you could. Topiramate works well in preventing migraine but some people experience a lot of side effects. You will only find out how well it works for you if you try it, and the same applies to side effects.

The specialist nurse has suggested I use topiramate for
migraine. What sort of side effects can I expect?

There are many different side effects that you might experience but the commonest tend to be paraesthesia (e.g. 'pins and needles' or prickling sensation) and sleep disturbance. In some people there are mood changes and emotional disturbances including anxiety, nervousness and depression. The most notable side effect is that it can cause weight loss; it is the only preventative migraine drug that has weight loss rather than weight gain listed as a side effect.

Some people experience few or no side effects; others who have mild side effects feel that the benefit is worth it. The only way to know is to try it.

It has been suggested that I try topiramate for my migraine.
What sort of dose do I need to take?

The usual dose for migraine prevention is 50 mg twice a day. Some people notice a benefit below this dose, and others need to get up to this dose. I usually start people on the 15 mg capsules, increasing the dose by 15 mg every two weeks to minimise the development of side effects, and ideally stop at the lowest dose needed to produce an effect.

I have just started topiramate but have been getting some funny sensations affecting my hands and feet. Is that normal?

This is one of the recognised side effects of topiramate and in that sense is normal. Only you can decide if the benefit you are getting from your topiramate is worth the side effects you are experiencing.

I've tried Epilim (sodium valproate) and topiramate with limited benefit. I have been reading on the internet about gabapentin and levetiracetam. Can you tell me anything about them?

Gabapentin is an AED that is used in treating epilepsy and chronic pain problems, such as back and neck pain and even neuralgia. There is some evidence to suggest that it can help some people reduce the number of migraine attacks that they experience. There are a range of side effects that you may experience; they include nausea and vomiting, diarrhoea, dizziness, drowsiness, fatigue, paraesthesia as well as some mood and emotional changes.

Levetiracetam is used mainly in epilepsy but some studies suggest that it can help in reducing migraine frequency. More studies are planned so, if you have had little or no benefit from other drugs, it is worth trying levetiracetam. There are a range of side effects associated with levetiracetam; they include drowsiness and dizziness, less commonly nausea, diarrhoea, emotional changes and double vision.

My GP has suggested I should take the antidepressant amitriptyline to stop my headache, but I am not depressed and don't want to take it. Why has he suggested it?

Although amitriptyline was developed to treat depression, it has also been used successfully to treat chronic pain – and, of course, headache is a form of chronic pain. If you view taking the drug as a way of stabilising the way your brain responds, it makes a little more sense! By raising your migraine threshold, it should reduce the chance of a migraine being triggered.

I have been taking amitriptyline but have found that if I take more than 20 mg I am too sleepy to get up in the morning. It seems to be easing my migraines, though, so is there anything I can do?

That rather depends on what time you actually take the amitriptyline. If you are having difficulty waking in the morning, try taking it 12 hours before you want to get up. If that doesn't work, you could try a similar drug called imipramine, which may cause you few or no side effects.

I have been given amitriptyline for my migraines but my sister was given imipramine. Is it any better?

That is not an easy question to answer, as it rather depends on what you mean by 'better'. If amitriptyline causes you to experience side effects, imipramine may suit you better. If the amitriptyline does not reduce the number of headache days you get, imipramine might suit you better. 'Better' is really what works for you.

Why do antidepressants and epilepsy drugs work in migraine when they were designed for such different problems in the first place?

I am not sure that anyone can really answer that question. Both types or 'classes' of drug are designed to have an effect on the brain, and both migraine and epilepsy are conditions that are caused by brain changes. Anything that can stabilise the brain's response and prevent these changes from occurring will prevent events happening, be they an epileptic or a migraine attack.

*I am a little curious as my specialist nurse says that
antidepressants will help my migraines but amitriptyline
and similar drugs have always made me feel really drowsy.
Is there any other sort of antidepressant that I can take that
has fewer side effects?*

Amitriptyline is one of the tricyclic antidepressants (TCAD) group
or class of drugs. Imipramine, dosulepin and nortriptyline are all
TCADs. Different people react differently to different drugs, and it may
be that with others you will not feel as drowsy as with one of the ones
you have tried already.

There is another type of antidepressant, collectively referred to as
selective serotonin re-uptake inhibitors (SSRIs), that is not associated
with the same sort of side effects as TCADs but there is no good evidence that these drugs are helpful in the management of migraine.

PREVENTATIVE DRUG TREATMENT FOR CLUSTER HEADACHE

*I have been told that I have episodic cluster headache.
What is the best way to stop the cluster episode?*

The cluster can be stopped, for some people, by taking a short
course of high-dose oral steroids. 'High' means about 60 mg,
ideally as an enteric-coated tablet, taken for two weeks. An 'enteric-
coated' tablet is one that has a coating that allows the drug to pass
through the stomach and arrive in the small intestine where it is
released and absorbed into the bloodstream. Preventing the drug from
being released in the stomach prevents any side effects such as heartburn, indigestion and possibly stomach ulcers.

My specialist says that I should take a high-dose course of
steroids but I am concerned about side effects. Should I be?

A ny drug can cause side effects, and the side effects will vary
according to the drug you use. You and your doctor choose a
drug because of the potential it has to fix or cure your symptoms. The
challenge with drugs that might cause significant side effects is how
good they are at curing your problem . . . and how bad your problem
is in the first place.

Steroids can cause symptoms of heartburn and indigestion and
even an ulcer. They can also lead to aches in the muscles and thin-
ning of the bones such as osteoporosis and possibly even fractures of
some bones. They can cause bone death (necrosis) of parts of bones
such as the head of the femur, or hip bone.

Who gets these side effects, how often they occur and whether they
occur at all is impossible to predict. The decision to take a drug can be
a difficult one that you should make in discussion with your doctor.

If I decide to take steroids for my cluster headache, can I just
stop them when they've had their effect?

T he only way to find out whether you can just stop them, or should
gradually reduce them, is to try it out and see what happens.
Some people find that they can simply stop their steroids once they
have completed their course and they do not get a flare-up of their
cluster headache. Others find that they have to reduce the dose slowly
over a week or two in order to be sure they have completely sup-
pressed the attack. A slow reduction of steroids is best with the higher
doses of steroids.

I have taken steroids and they stopped my cluster headache within a few days but every time I stop taking them the headache comes back within a few weeks. What can I do?

If the steroids work but the headache comes back again, it may be that you need a slightly higher dose, or you need to take it for a little longer or you need to think about using a second drug to prevent the headache from coming back when you stop the steroids. Contact your doctor about this to discuss the options that are available to you.

The steroids work really well in stopping my cluster headache but I get quite bad indigestion with them. Is there anything I can do?

Yes, there is. If steroids really are that effective, taking a drug to protect your stomach will prevent the indigestion from developing. The drug usually used to achieve this is in a class called *proton pump inhibitors*; the most commonly used one is omeprazole. Talk to your doctor about the problem to find the best solution for you.

I have cluster headache and the specialist has suggested that I need to take a preventative drug as he feels it is the chronic form. What are my options?

There are a variety of drugs that can be used but the research evidence suggests the best one is the drug called verapamil. Verapamil is a calcium channel blocker that is usually used to treat certain heart arrhythmias, angina and hypertension.

Other drugs have been tried, such as Epilim (sodium valproate), topiramate and lithium. Studies that looked at their effectiveness have met with varying degrees of success.

The specialist has told me that I need to increase the dose of verapamil but will have to have an ECG every time I increase the dose. Why?

Verapamil can be very effective in managing cluster headache. The drug has an effect on how the electrical impulses pass through the heart: when used in a dose appropriate to treat cluster headache, this effect can be significant. Doing a heart tracing – the ECG – allows the nurse or specialist to make sure that no abnormal change is happening to how the heart is working.

My GP says that the dose of verapamil suggested by the specialist is too high. If that is the case, why has the specialist suggested it?

Drugs are licensed for use in specific conditions and the doses used have been confirmed in a variety of drug trials. It is uncommon for those drugs to be used at maximum doses.

When you use these drugs in specialist settings and the normal, more standard, doses do not seem to have the desired effect, the boundaries can be stretched a little. If your ECG is normal, your specialist will suggest pushing the dose up a bit in the hope that this will stop your cluster headache; then the dose can be reduced to more normal levels as soon as possible.

Verapamil doesn't work for my cluster headache, so what else can I try?

You say that verapamil does not work for your cluster headache but you do not say what sort of dose you have used and how long you took it. You need to increase the dose of verapamil to your maximum tolerated dose, one that does not cause side effects, or the maximum recommended dose for the drug itself.

You also need to take the verapamil for long enough to work. It usually takes verapamil two weeks at any one dose to produce its effect, and if it is effective then it should be continued for long enough. How long that is depends on how long your episode of cluster headache usually lasts. I usually suggest two weeks after you would have expected the bout to end normally.

If verapamil still does not work, another possibility for you to try could be an anti-epilepsy drug, such as sodium valproate or topiramate or lithium.

I know that anti-epilepsy drugs help in migraine, but can they help my cluster headache?

Yes, they can. Some scientific studies have looked at different antiepilepsy drugs and how effective they might be in preventing cluster headache. The degree of effectiveness is variable but, if all else fails, nothing ventured nothing gained.

If I go ahead and try an anti-epilepsy drug, how do I decide which one to take?

Choosing a drug is about trying to decide how effective it will be and what sort of side effects it can have. If one anti-epilepsy drug (AED) doesn't work, trying an alternative is worth considering. Epilim (sodium valproate) and topiramate are likely to be the first choices that your doctor will suggest, on the basis of current evidence.

I currently take lithium for my cluster headache. Why do I have to have a blood test every three months?

It is important to make sure that you are not taking too much lithium, and this can be checked with a blood test. Lithium has been known to lead to an underactive thyroid gland and thyroid function should be checked regularly, initially every three months and then, once the dose is stable, every six to twelve months. The blood test will check how much lithium you have in your blood, and check how your thyroid gland is working.

I'm going to be taking lithium. How long do I need to take it?

Using a preventative drug for cluster headache is about suppressing the bout of episodic cluster headache. The length of each bout tends to vary from person to person, so how long you take the lithium will vary accordingly. If your bout lasts three months, take it for four months; if it lasts for six months, take it for seven or eight months.

Some people develop a more chronic (long-lasting) form of cluster headache and they have to take preventative treatment on a more permanent basis, possibly forever.

PREVENTATIVE DRUG TREATMENT FOR TENSION-TYPE HEADACHE

How can I stop my tension-type headaches from becoming migraines?

Tension-type headache does not really become migraine, but I think I know what you mean. It is possible that your migraine seems to start with a sore aching neck before your more normal migraine headache begins. What you have is a 'mixed picture' headache. You get migraine some of the time and tension-type headache some of the time, and sometimes one starts just before the other.

The best way to stop the tension-type headache becoming migraine is to stop the tension-type headache happening in the first place by keeping your headache threshold as high as you can. If you get a mild headache, think about the things that you can do to ease the symptoms. If they happen only every now and again, simple painkillers are a good idea, but if you have quite frequent headaches then you may need to think about trying a preventative drug.

My GP has suggested that I should take an antidepressant rather than a painkiller for my tension-type headache. Why?

Tension-type headache is often episodic – that is to say, it happens occasionally, every now and again, with no headache symptoms in between. The more frequent your tension-type headache, the more often you might be tempted to take painkillers for it. And the more often you take painkillers, the greater the risk of developing medication overuse headache. Your GP has suggested that you take an antidepressant to try to ease your headache while avoiding the use of painkillers; it should also reduce the chance of medication overuse headache developing and allow your tension-type headache to settle.

The nurse has said 'don't treat the low-impact headache'. But if I can't take a painkiller, what can I do for my headache?

The nurse has suggested that you avoid treating a low-impact headache because she wants to minimise the risk of your developing a medication overuse headache.

There are a variety of things you can do to help your tension-type headache. They include massage, using a wheat bag or other source of local heat, increasing your water intake, having a soak in the bath or any other way that helps you to relax and unwind.

For more ideas about self-help, look at Chapters 7 and 8.

The specialist has suggested that I take a drug usually used to treat epilepsy for my tension-type headache. How is that going to help?

An anti-epilepsy drug (AED) can be used to treat a variety of chronic pain conditions. Tension-type headache is a chronic pain and can respond well to an AED. Although how it works isn't fully understood, the fact is that it can work and is certainly worth trying. The goal is to reduce the total number of headache days, and taking medication is one way of doing it.

I don't like taking painkillers and I don't want to take a preventative drug, so what do I do about my chronic tension-type headache?

You could start with diet and lifestyle changes (for more information on self-help, see Chapter 7). If that doesn't work, you might want to consider a variety of complementary therapies, such as aromatherapy and massage to help you relax. Yoga or reflexology might help, and acupuncture or osteopathy could make a difference. (Complementary therapies are discussed in Chapter 8.)

13 | Tackling medication overuse headache

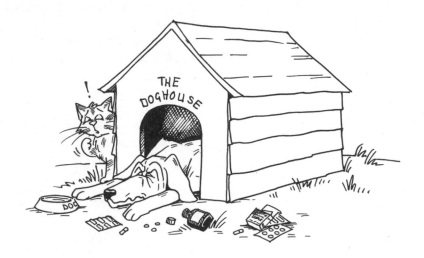

Medication overuse headache (MOH) is challenging to treat because, first and foremost, it is about stopping taking the painkillers. Doing this successfully means finding the strategy relevant to you, as an individual; what works for one person may not necessarily work for another. In most instances you will need to rely on the help and support of your GP or practice nurse throughout this process, as headache clinics and specialist nurses are not a readily accessible resource. As you read through this chapter you may have to substitute the word 'nurse' with whoever you are using as your support person; realistically that could be anyone, although you will need the assistance of a GP if you need prescribed medication or a sick note.

MOH is where an occasional headache becomes a daily or near-daily headache. It is a headache associated with the uncritical use of painkillers, increasingly frequent use of painkillers and the use of stronger and stronger painkillers to treat headache symptoms. Research has shown that 71% of people with MOH started with migraine alone, 14% started with tension-type headache alone and 15% had a mixed picture headache of migraine and tension-type headache.

STOPPING THE PAINKILLERS – THE FIRST STEP BACK TO EPISODIC HEADACHE

My GP has told me about medication overuse headache and how to stop it but I just cannot imagine getting through the day without any painkillers. How am I going to cope?

Coping is about getting back in control of your headache symptoms. It means swapping your daily headache for a headache that occurs every now and again. Coping is about changing what you do in response to your headache. It is about putting strategies or 'cushions' in place to help you manage your headache without taking a painkiller. The cushions you need will be unique to you and how you cope will be unique to you. There is always a way – you just have to find out what it is. There is no right or wrong way – what this chapter does is offer you ideas and make suggestions.

The specialist has said I need to stop taking my painkillers but how can I do it?

You need to find your own way. You can either stop all of your painkillers immediately or gradually reduce them to the point where you stop using them. The best way is the way that will work for you. If you are taking strong painkillers, especially if they contain codeine and caffeine, it is probably better to stop them by gradually reducing the number you take to try to minimise the 'rebound' withdrawal symptoms you might experience. (See also the next answer.)

I am in the process of trying to stop taking my painkillers. The specialist nurse kept talking about withdrawal symptoms – what does she mean?

When you stop taking your painkillers you can expect to experience symptoms that occur as a direct consequence. This 'rebound' effect is inevitable: the type and severity of these symptoms are unpredictable and vary from person to person and from headache to headache. If your primary headache is migraine, many of your rebound symptoms will be similar to those of your migraine – including headache, nausea, vomiting, light sensitivity, mood swings, irritability and sleep disturbance. If your primary headache is tension-type headache (TTH), your symptoms will resemble those of TTH, including worsening headache, irritability and sleep disturbance.

I am worried because I use co-codamol for my headache. I only take two a day, but I have to take them every day. Will that make it harder to stop?

The only answer I can offer is that it might. Codeine is an addictive drug. Co-codamol comes in a dose of 8 mg or 30 mg of codeine mixed with 500 mg of paracetamol. The higher the strength of co-codamol you take, the harder it might be to stop. The more you take each day the harder it might be to stop. Many over-the-counter painkillers contain some codeine as well, so you need to check just how much codeine you are actually taking.

I take co-codamol and have been told that the best way to stop, because of the codeine, is to gradually reduce the tablets. Why is this so?

Stopping codeine causes side effects, and in someone with medication overdose headache stopping painkillers abruptly may lead to 'rebound' symptoms. Stopping painkillers when you have medication overuse headache is always difficult, and success often depends on minimising the effect of withdrawal. Codeine is an addictive drug, and reducing the dose of co-codamol gradually also reduces the sort of side effects you might experience in stopping the codeine.

I have been taking co-codamol, up to eight a day, but not necessarily every day. The specialist nurse has suggested that I gradually reduce the dose of codeine, but how gradually is gradually?

How quickly or slowly you reduce your tablets depends on exactly how many you take and what strength the codeine is. If you are taking 30-mg-strength tablets, especially if you are taking two tablets each time, I suggest that you take an 8 mg instead of one of the 30 mg tablets. This way you gradually reduce the amount of codeine you take each time, and then you can gradually reduce the total number of doses each day.

It can be difficult to know over how many days you make this dose reduction – it will often be decided according to the sort of symptoms you experience. Only you can make that decision, and your specialist nurse can help you as you do so.

My friend takes Syndol for her headaches, and she has suggested that as they help her a little I should try them for my headaches. Is that a good idea?

If you have frequent headaches, or have MOH, swapping one painkiller for another is not really a good idea. Any painkiller, including Syndol, Solpadeine (both with paracetamol) or Nurofen (ibuprofen), has the ability to lead to MOH if taken on more than three or four days in the week, and therefore should be used only infrequently to treat headache.

If the headache is going to get worse when I stop the painkillers, what can I do for the headache? I have to be able to get through the day somehow.

The only way to break the MOH cycle is to take no painkillers at all for at least six to eight weeks. If you take any painkillers at all during this 'washout' phase, it may make it less likely that the headaches will improve.

Not taking painkillers when the headache gets bad is not easy. You may need to think about taking time off work (your GP should be able to help with a sick note) or you may need to think about other medication used to treat chronic pain, which could help reduce the headache you experience. By taking something else, a preventative drug every day, you may be able to ease or stop or headache and avoid the need for painkillers. This will make it easier for you to successfully stop the painkillers and allow your headache to become episodic and infrequent again.

For more information on preventative drugs, see Chapter 12.

I know that my headaches may well get worse when I stop my painkillers. What else can I expect?

It is always difficult to know what will happen, because everyone is different. The possible symptoms include nausea and sometimes vomiting, sensitivity to light, feeling bad-tempered and irritable, getting mood swings and having difficulty sleeping. It is unlikely that you will experience all of these but you could experience any one of them at some time during your 'washout'.

The clinic has said that I can't take any painkillers for at least six weeks. That seems an awfully long time. Do I really have to wait that long?

Medication overuse headache is always difficult to treat. Success can be achieved only if you take no painkillers at all. The longer you can avoid taking painkillers, the more likely that your headache will improve. Your specialist has suggested six weeks as the starting point but will probably encourage you to carry on for another week or two so that your total washout is for eight weeks, and perhaps even longer. It depends on how quickly your headache improves. If your headache is slow to respond, prolonging the washout is the best way to go. Some people find that they notice a dramatic improvement in a week or two whereas others may need as long as ten or twelve weeks; everyone is different and there is no real way of predicting how quickly or slowly things will change.

It is not easy but try hard to stick to it, because it is the only way. Remember to ask all your friends and family to help; that way you are more likely to succeed.

COPING WITHOUT PAINKILLERS

I get a headache every day and the last time I tried to stop the painkillers the headache got so bad I had to start taking them again. I have to go to work and the only way to get through the day is to take the tablets. I just don't think I can stop; what can I do?

Stopping painkillers is never easy. If your headache started off as migraine, the 'rebound' symptoms can be quite severe and be similar to the severity of migraine attacks themselves. The only way to completely break the medication overuse headache cycle is to stop using painkillers completely, no matter how bad your headache gets.

To be successful you need support. This can come from your friends, your family or your work colleagues or it can come from medication that is not a painkiller but can help the pain from your headache. Your doctor or nurse will encourage you to seek help from those around you. It is about putting a strategy in place that can help you not only now but also in the future.

You need to consider all the options and decide exactly what you must do to reduce the chance of a headache developing. finding a way of not taking the painkiller is about changing how you react and respond to pain or finding a way of stopping the pain happening in the first place.

For information about self-help options, see Chapter 7. You might also find useful information in Chapter 8, on complementary therapies.

I have young children and there are times when the headache gets so bad that I have to take something for it. Even though it does not get rid of the pain, it means I can look after the children until my husband gets home. What can I do if I can't take the painkillers?

The challenge you have is that with medication overuse headache you must break the cycle. To break the cycle you have to stop taking the painkillers *completely* during the washout phase. To do that you have to do away with all the circumstances or situations that will provoke you into taking a tablet. You have to find a way of doing this, whatever it takes.

If the barrier to stopping the painkillers is 'who's going to look after the children?' you need to find a time when it won't be a barrier. This could mean arranging for a friend or family member to look after the children, so that you can concentrate on stopping the painkillers. You might need only a short period of time (a few days) or it could take a little longer (a week or two); there is no way of knowing just how long this it will be. It is one of those times when you really do have to take each day as it comes. To stop successfully, you need to plan carefully and ask for help and support from people around you.

For more information on self-help, look at Chapter 7. And see also the next two answers.

The nurse at the clinic has been talking to me about different drugs I can use during the washout phase. How do I decide which one to take?

Choosing which drug to use is not an easy or straightforward decision. Some are automatically ruled out if you have specific medical conditions, such as asthma, so this is a 'negative choice'. Some are automatically chosen because you have another medical condition that would benefit from a particular drug, so a 'positive choice'. Some are chosen because of their possible side effects: sedation if you need to sleep, weight loss if you could do with losing some weight.

When the nurse sees you she will talk to you about the different drugs available and deciding which best meets your needs or suits you. There is no way of predicting which choice is the right one; there is the one that works for you but it is not always possible to choose the right one first time. Sometimes trial and error is the only way to move things forward.

The nurse has said that there are tablets I can take to help the pain that are not painkillers. She said that they are antidepressants but I am not depressed. Why should I take antidepressants?

Medication overuse headache can be seen as a form of chronic pain, and there is range of drugs that are used to help chronic pain that are not painkillers. One of these is a group of drugs called tricyclic antidepressants. Stopping this headache is about stopping the painkillers, and if taking a tricyclic antidepressant will help you do that, it is worth thinking about.

It is another one of those 'nothing ventured, nothing gained' situations. It could make the difference between taking back control and just not getting there, so why not give it a try?

Why can't I just take prophylaxis to make the headaches go away?

Prophylaxis can help, but if you have medication overuse headache you have to stop the painkillers as well. Understanding why this is essential is often difficult. It just doesn't seem to make sense that tablets designed to stop pain should apparently cause it. Perhaps I can explain it here.

Pain is felt when a receptor in the brain is stimulated. What happens with medication overuse headache is that the receptors get reset and, instead of being 'switched off' by the painkiller, are actually kept 'switched on'. Pain is a response to a stimulus or irritant. When you have medication overuse headache, the receptor is so sensitive that it takes very little to produce a pain response. The only way to reset the receptor is to stop the painkiller.

Painkillers and triptans seem to wind things up, making the nerves 'irritable', whereas preventative drugs help calm this response down and stabilise the nerve so that pain is felt less often and the response is at a lower and more normal threshold.

How can I make sure I succeed? I have tried to stop painkillers before but it just got too hard.

Success is about how badly you want to succeed and who else you get to help and support you while you go through the washout phase. It may be that you need to arrange some time off work, or get help with the children. Think about what will be happening during the washout period. Take positive steps and make positive choices and decisions. If you couldn't do it on your own before, ask for help and support this time. People will help if they know you need it and why.

The nurse has said that I cannot take any painkillers during my 'washout'. Why not?

The receptors in the brain have been reset by your taking regular painkillers, and as a result it takes very little to stimulate the receptor to send signals telling that you are in pain. The receptors have to learn to respond correctly rather than over-enthusiastically. The washout means exactly that, it is a washing out of the receptors so that they respond more appropriately in the future.

My nurse at the clinic has said that I can call her any time. Will that really make a difference?

Yes, it can. Changing what you do is always difficult. It is easier to change if you have someone to help you. In some ways stopping your painkiller is like trying to deal with an addiction to anything, such as nicotine or alcohol. You need all the help you can get, so grab the opportunity with both hands! If you feel the need to take a painkiller, phone the nurse and talk to her instead.

Is there a good time to stop taking painkillers? I really want my headache to get better but it just seems so hard.

There is a good time to stop, and that is the time when you feel that you can do it successfully. This may take a little planning and thinking about. It means making sure that you have all the help and support in place that you feel you need.

I'm not getting a headache every day now, but I'm still getting some bad days when I have to go to bed. When are the headaches going to stop?

It is always difficult to know exactly what will happen when you stop the painkillers. The background headache should improve slowly with time. This means that you will shift slowly from a daily or near-daily headache to an episodic headache. The episodic headache is the one that you started with before your headache increased in frequency as a result of your use of painkillers.

If this headache is bad enough to send you to bed, it is probably migraine. But you still need to complete your washout because the longer you can keep going the better. Eventually all that you will be left with is the occasional bad headache, probably migraine, which you can then treat.

What happens if the headaches don't get better when I stop taking the painkillers?

It would be unusual for the headaches to not change at all. You should notice a reduction in the total number of headache days that you get. There will be a gradual shift from daily headache, to fewer headache days, to no dull aching background headache to just the occasional migraine. It is unlikely that the headaches will stop completely but they should significantly reduce in frequency so that they become manageable and treatable.

If your headaches do not improve, you should continue not taking painkillers but think about taking a preventative drug. This would help control your headache and make it easier to stay off the painkillers. It may be that you need the preventative drug to 'switch off' the nerve response completely.

I have done really well and have stopped all my painkillers. That nagging background headache has gone but I still need to treat the migraine. I am worried that if I start treating the migraine my daily headache will come back. What should I do?

There is always a chance that your daily headache might return. Your migraine is a high-impact headache that needs treating. The best thing to do is to find the most effective acute treatment that gets rid of your migraine attack and makes sure that it stays away. This is called a 'sustained pain-free response'.

What you need to look out for are shifts in how your attack responds to your acute treatment. If your migraine seems to become less responsive, takes longer to settle and recurs more often, you need to be aware that the medication overuse headache may be coming back. If the number of headache days starts to increase, you may need to think about prophylaxis. Prophylaxis, or prevention, is about reducing the total number of headache days so that you don't have too many days taking acute treatments.

STOPPING TAKING TRIPTANS

My doctor says I have to stop taking my triptan every day but he wants me to take another tablet every day instead. I'm happy taking my sumatriptan when I need it, as it takes away my pain and allows me to get on with my life. I think what my doctor is suggesting could lead to lots of side effects and my headache will get worse. What do you think?

It is my opinion that, if you have to take sumatriptan every day, you have a medication overuse headache – that is, a *triptan rebound headache*. The headache develops as the effect of the triptan wears off, stimulating you to take another dose of the triptan; it does work but in this case is actually responsible for the headache developing the next day even though it seems to 'fix' the problem in the short term.

The only way to stop this rebound headache from happening is to stop the triptan. Yes, your symptoms will get worse in the short term but you will then go back to an episodic migraine rather than a daily migraine-like headache. I encourage you to take a preventative drug in the short term to reduce the severity and impact of the withdrawal symptoms and possibly even in the medium term to minimise the number of headache days that you get, reducing the chance of developing rebound headache symptoms again in the future.

I use a triptan to treat my migraine. My GP says that I am taking too many but I have to take the triptan or the migraine doesn't settle. Is my GP right?

Your GP is probably right. The threshold for what is called 'triptan rebound' is about 8 to 10 triptans a month, and this applies to any triptan. If you are taking more than 10, it is almost certain that your triptan is contributing to your headache. Headache recurrence when treating migraine is not unusual and occurs in 25–50% of attacks. Repeating the dose is the right thing to do provided you get migraines only every now and again. The more frequent your migraines, the more headache days you have and the more days you take an acute treatment. The shift from episodic headache to medication overuse headache occurs with remarkable ease in some individuals!

Why does my migraine seem to come back? I am taking a triptan every day now. If I don't take it early the headache just gets worse instead of better.

It sounds as if you have a triptan rebound headache. The headache often comes back at the same time every day. The brain's pain receptors stop working properly, the headache creeps back and you feel you have to take another triptan – it becomes a vicious circle. It is just the same as getting medication overuse headache when taking ordinary painkillers.

COPING WITHOUT TRIPTANS

I only take my triptan because the headache gets really bad. I just don't know how I am going to avoid taking one for at least six weeks. What else can I do?

Stopping triptans is never easy because the rebound headaches tend to be quite significant. Careful planning as to *when* you stop is as crucial to success as the *how*. Using preventative drugs as a routine measure is recommended, which, as always, is a balance between effectiveness, side effects and possible risks.

Is there anything I can do to make it easier to stop taking my triptan?

Everyone is different in how they set about making such a significant change. You need to think carefully about potential triggers and stresses that contribute to your migraines. Also, make sure that you are in the best possible situation with all the support you need in place.

The specialist nurse has suggested that I may need to be admitted to hospital to stop my triptan. Why might this happen?

The nurse has probably suggested this so that you are given the best possible chance of success. In hospital you will have none of the sorts of stresses and hassles that would occur at home. It also means that there will be people around who can help with any rebound symptoms you get and offer appropriate drug treatment if needed.

The specialist nurse has suggested that I take some beta-blockers when I stop taking my triptan. Can they help?

I have found that beta-blockers seem to work well in relieving or easing the rebound symptoms when triptans are stopped. I usually recommend a 160 mg dose of propranolol as a slow-release preparation, which is taken just once a day.

However, if you have asthma or a history of asthma, beta-blockers are not an option for you. If that is the case, the nurse will discuss other preventative drugs with you. (See also Chapter 12.)

I have been told to expect nausea and vomiting as well as the chance that the headache may get worse before it gets better. Is there any way to ease those symptoms?

Research offers a variety of options, although none of them gives an absolute guarantee of success. The suggestions that I offer are based on the published evidence base and the experience we have built up at the headache clinic in York.

I suggest using metoclopramide or domperidone to ease the nausea and vomiting, and often suggest using diazepam as well. The diazepam is optional, but I usually encourage patients who have been overusing triptans for months, rather than days and weeks, to consider it. Diazepam is helpful if you are likely to get mood swings, irritability or sleep disturbance when stopping your medication – which in my experience is most likely when stopping triptans.

I would normally suggest using this mix of drugs for seven to ten days to ease the most severe 'rebound' symptoms.

I have stopped my triptans and feel that the propranolol has helped. How long should I take the propranolol after stopping my triptan?

Well done for having successfully stopped your triptans – not an easy thing to do. If the propranolol is helping to ease your symptoms, I suggest continuing to take it for a minimum of eight weeks. There is no absolute rule to help you decide how much longer after that you should carry on taking the propranolol.

There are times when it is a good idea to take the propranolol for three months; sometimes it may be longer. The decision has to be taken on a day-by-day or week-by-week basis.

I had a lot of rebound symptoms when I stopped taking my triptan and was given diazepam and metoclopramide. The nurse has said I should stop taking them now. Are my symptoms likely to return?

Diazepam and metoclopramide should be used only in the very short term and I tend to suggest using them for no longer than the first seven to ten days. This provides cover for the most severe symptoms experienced in the first few days after the triptans have been stopped.

The most severe symptoms should not return, and are most commonly associated with stopping triptans. Your headache symptoms will take longer to settle and this is why you will be encouraged to take preventative medication. If you are already on a preventative drug, it makes sense to carry on taking it in the short term and possibly in the medium term.

A friend of mine was given steroids when she stopped taking her triptans. It has not been suggested to me. Why not?

It is difficult to give you a simple answer to that question. There has been some research looking at what drugs offer the best way of easing or completely alleviating the symptoms associated with triptan withdrawal. One piece of research looked at using high-dose oral steroids, at a dose of 60 to 80 mg taken over the first three days that no triptans are taken. The results of the published trials were not very conclusive, so it is an option that tends not to be used as much now.

I can't take beta-blockers because I have asthma. What are my options to try to ease my withdrawal symptoms?

You can try any of the standard migraine-preventative drugs, including tricyclic antidepressants and anti-epilepsy drugs. There is no 'right' choice. The decision-making is no different from that with the options discussed in Chapter 12.

14 | Children and headaches

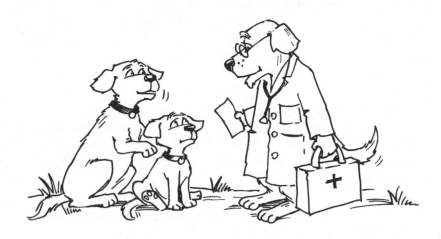

Children can get the same sorts of headaches as adults. There are times when diagnosing the problem is harder but patience and listening to the parents and the child are usually rewarded. The criteria for making a diagnosis have been changed and modified over time to better reflect the reality of headache in childhood.

Non-drug treatments are often underrated as a way of improving headache in childhood: relatively simple changes can have a dramatic effect on the frequency of headaches. Choosing drugs to treat the acute headache can also be difficult because of drug licensing rules. The same range of drugs can be used for children but there must be careful discussion resulting in informed consent involving the parents or guardian or other responsible adult and the child. Similar choices and decisions have to be made with preventative drugs as well.

DIAGNOSING HEADACHE IN CHILDREN

How will the doctor be able to tell that my child has migraine?

The diagnosis of migraine in children, as in adults, is made on the basis of the International Headache Society (IHS) classification, which uses a set of criteria that need to be met. Diagnosis can be more difficult in children, as the symptoms may be short-lasting and may not always occur every time. The child may not associate the symptoms with the headache, or have the ability to describe them.

The symptoms must be sensitive enough and specific enough to make the diagnosis of migraine. *Sensitivity* is about choosing the symptoms that discriminate and separate the different types of headaches accurately enough. *Specificity* is about choosing the symptoms that are precise and limited enough to separate the different types of headache. The higher the sensitivity and specificity of a set of symptoms, the more accurate and reliable the diagnosis of migraine compared with any other headache.

The IHS criteria for diagnosing migraine in a child are:

- The headache attack lasts from 2 to 48 hours

- The headache has at least two of the following:

  – it is one-sided

  – has a throbbing quality

  – is of moderate to severe intensity

  – is aggravated by routine physical activity

- The child has at least one of the following:

  – nausea and/or vomiting

  – sensitivity to light or sound

I get migraine and find it hard enough to describe my symptoms. How can I get my daughter, who is eight, to explain hers to our GP?

It is difficult to describe symptoms that you are experiencing to someone else, but do the best you can with prompting from the doctor. Your GP will, with time and patience, be able to get a feel for what is happening to your daughter. You can help by describing what you see happening when your daughter is having her attack or you could ask your daughter to draw a picture to show how it affects her.

There are some points your GP needs to be aware of, because migraine in children can be quite different from that experienced by adults. The headache, if present, is often much shorter than in adults. Nausea and vomiting may be more dominant than the headache.

Migraine sufferers are often very pale and quiet during an attack. This may be the best clue, rather than a description of what is happening.

I'm worried about my grandson. He doesn't complain of headache but every now and again goes really pale and just curls up on the sofa rocking back and forth. He's like this for a few hours and then bounces back, right as rain. I remember his mum having similar problems and now she has migraine. Could this be the start of migraine in him?

Yes, it could. What effect or impact the symptoms have is often the best guide to what is happening. Going pale and looking ill may be the only symptom of migraine in young children. How he seems, looks or behaves may be the only clue you have that he might be having a migraine. Headache does not always occur, or if it does may not be particularly severe.

The diagnosis of migraine is made on the basis that the same sequence of events recurs over time, and follows the same pattern on each occasion. This is called 'being stereotypical'.

I think my son has migraine but my GP says it doesn't last long enough. Is he right?

Migraine headache in children tends to be shorter than in adults, and generally tends to be shorter the younger the child. The headache may last as little as 1 or 2 hours and perhaps no longer than 24 to 48 hours. Making the diagnosis is not just about how long the headache lasts but also the other associated symptoms of migraine such as being sensitive to light or feeling sick. An accurate diagnosis is about getting a feel for the balance of different symptoms and how they come together – the need for high sensitivity and specificity.

My son keeps having bouts of gastroenteritis, or at least that's what I thought they were. I took him to see our GP because he often has two or three days off school with diarrhoea and vomiting. The GP has suggested that it could be migraine. Could it?

It is certainly a possibility, especially if no other cause can be found. Children experience migraine in different ways and this sort of episodic bouts of illness is consistent with a possible diagnosis of migraine, especially if he looks pale, has some abdominal pain and is very quiet and withdrawn. If your GP has ruled out any infective or other cause then migraine is quite possible.

I thought the pain of migraine had to be one-sided and not on both sides. I am sure my daughter has migraine but she gets pain on both sides of her head. Could it still be migraine?

One-sided pain is only one possible symptom in the diagnosis of migraine. The pain can occur on both sides, the diagnosis depending on what the pain feels like and some or all of the other associated symptoms. So it could still be migraine despite the fact that pain occurs on both sides of your daughter's head. Remember that migraine does not follow all of the rules all of the time, and headaches in children are the most unpredictable of all.

> *I think my daughter has migraine but when we went to the GP she found it difficult to describe her pain. How important is that in deciding what sort of headache she has?*

Describing pain is never easy but the severity or impact of the pain tends to offer a better clue to the diagnosis. Making the diagnosis of migraine is not just about describing the pain but asking about all the symptoms that are associated with migraine as well.

> *I took my son to see a specialist and she said that he has a migraine variant. What does that mean?*

A *migraine variant* tends to be a form of migraine in which the headache tends to be less significant and the other migrainous symptoms more prominent. There are three different types currently within the International Headache Society classification:

- cyclical vomiting
- abdominal migraine
- benign paroxysmal vertigo of childhood

It is felt that although these types are not migraine they do occur in childhood and may herald the development of migraine in later years. (See the next few answers for more information about these types.)

> *What is cyclical vomiting? I was reading about it on a website and wondered if that is what my grandchild has. She has been admitted to hospital twice now with dehydration.*

Cyclical vomiting is a condition that is associated with intense nausea and vomiting, lasting for at least one hour and up to five days. The vomiting will occur several times an hour, for at least an hour. The child is often very pale and lethargic during an attack, and completely well between attacks.

Our GP says that my daughter has 'abdominal migraine'. I thought you had to have headache to have migraine, so what does she mean?

No, you don't have to have a headache to have migraine. In *abdominal migraine* there is abdominal pain that tends to last from 1 hour to 72 hours. I would expect your daughter to look pale, feel nauseated or vomit, and she would choose to avoid bright lights. These last symptoms are similar to those of migraine, which is why the condition is called abdominal migraine. (See also the next answer.)

The abdominal pain is a substitute for the head pain and tends to be moderate or severe in intensity. It can be dull or the child will describe it as 'sore'. The pain can be quite generalised or might be around the belly button (umbilicus).

I was told that I had abdominal migraine when I was a child but as I got older I seemed to get more and more headaches. Is that normal?

Yes, it is, or at least it can be. The consensus seems to be that, if you get abdominal migraine, you are likely to develop more typical migraine as you get older. There will be a shift from abdominal pain to headache with time.

I know what vertigo is like, but how can it be 'benign' when the symptoms are so horrid?

It is not particularly benign as an experience, but is benign in that there is no underlying 'sinister' or pathological cause. It affects young children and they become unsteady quite suddenly, grabbing on to any nearby object to stop themselves from falling over. They

234 MIGRAINE: ANSWERS AT YOUR FINGERTIPS

vomit, often profusely. If you look closely at the eyes you may see *nystagmus* – a jerking, side-to-side or up-and-down movement. The attacks occur repeatedly over several days before settling for a few weeks before recurring.

I used to get travel sickness as a child and now I have migraine. My son has started to get problems with travel sickness. Do you think he could develop migraine, too?

Yes, it is possible. Up to 40% of children with migraine have travel sickness. Migraine being triggered by travel may be a result of many different factors, including changed eating patterns, dehydration and flickering bright lights, to name a few.

For more information on triggers, see Chapter 7.

How on earth can my young son have a tension headache? He's only a child.

Anyone can get a tension-type headache, be it child or adult. The term is used to describe the particular mix of symptoms involved, not necessarily the cause.

A tension-type headache can be similar to migraine in some children because the migraine headache is often not as severe as in an adult. Tension-type headache is not associated with nausea or sensitivity to light and sound whereas migraine is. Moreover, the headache is more likely to occur on both sides, and to be of mild to moderate intensity rather than severe. It is more likely to be felt as a tightness or pressure than pulsing or throbbing. The headache can last for as little as half an hour or for several days.

My neighbour's teenage son has headaches that sound very like my cluster headache. Can children get cluster headache?

Yes, they can. Cluster headache is rare under the age of 10, but can occur for the first time at any age. It most commonly occurs for the first time between the ages of 20 and 40, with more men being affected than women.

My daughter seems to be getting a headache most days. She does not often have time off school but she always seems to have a headache by the time she gets home. What sort of headache could she have?

It is difficult to be sure, but daily headache is not migraine. It may be a tension-type headache or possibly a chronic daily headache or even a chronic tension-type headache. If she has been taking regular painkillers, it could also be a medication overuse headache. From what you have described so far, it is not possible to be sure.

I would look out for the usual diet and lifestyle things initially, such as regular meal patterns and a sensible fluid intake. It might be worth having a word with the teacher to see if there is anything your daughter is having problems with that she is not telling you.

What should I do if I am worried about my daughter's headaches? She seems to be getting them more often than ever before.

If you are worried about your daughter's headache, it would be sensible to go and have a chat to your GP. If your GP feels that your daughter's headaches fit neatly into a particular 'diagnostic box', he will offer appropriate advice for that type of headache. If he feels that your daughter's headache does not neatly fit into any 'box', she may be referred to a paediatrician or paediatric neurologist. Headaches can be difficult to assess, especially in children, even though they can get the same sorts of headaches as adults.

One of my friends at school seems to be taking lots of paracetamol. She says that she has to take them to stop her headache getting worse. Should I get her to talk to someone about it?

Yes, you should – the challenge will be to convince her that she needs to. The regular use of any painkiller to treat headache has the potential to cause a shift from occasional headache to daily headache that becomes less and less responsive to the treatment. If she is using paracetamol that often, it is quite possible that she has a medication overuse headache and needs to see her GP for help in stopping the paracetamol.

For more advice and information about medication overuse headache, read Chapter 13.

My son is getting what I thought were migraines but they seem to be happening more often. At what point should I take him to our GP?

You should take him if you are worried or concerned in any way. If you feel that there has been a significant change in how often he gets his migraine, an assessment by his GP will help rule out a potentially serious (or 'sinister') cause.

Your GP will want to know:

- if there are any new symptoms associated with his migraine
- if the symptoms have become more intense or dramatic
- if the headache is always on the same side or changes and swaps sides

The sorts of symptoms that cause concern are basically anything that is out of the ordinary and is different from anything that has been experienced before. If you are worried about it, do ask.

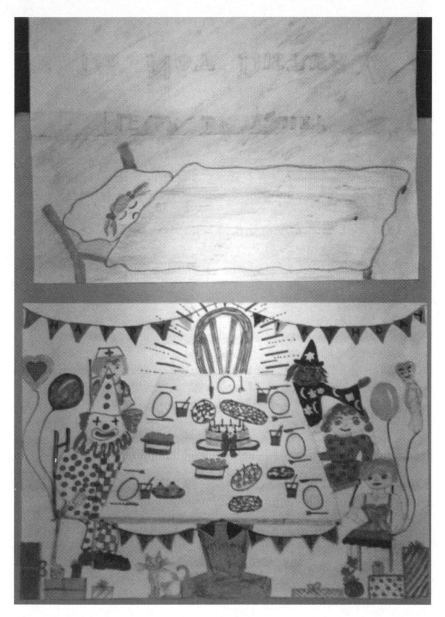

Plate 1 From the Migraine Art collection, reproduced by kind permission of the Migraine Action Association and Boehringer Ingelheim

How can I tell if the headaches my child is experiencing are sinister or not?

Sinister symptoms or 'red flags' are the same in children as in adults. A high temperature might suggest infection such as meningitis or encephalitis. 'Focal' symptoms such as weakness, pins and needles, numbness or other sensory changes might indicate a structural lesion in the brain. Fits could be a sign of a structural lesion or the start of epilepsy. A headache that rapidly increases in frequency and severity over days and weeks is more likely to cause concern than if the change occurs over months.

If you are worried or concerned about anything that happens, do ask your doctor for advice and assessment. Similarly, if there is a change in the pattern of symptoms that you feel is not quite right, ask about it.

My nephew has recently been diagnosed with a brain tumour. The headaches seemed to come on over a few weeks, and then he started to have fits. My eldest gets migraine, and I'm worried that she could have a brain tumour as well. What should I look out for with my own kids?

Migraine is much more common than a brain tumour. The longer the symptoms have been present, the less likely they are to be associated with a serious cause. Symptoms that swap sides are less likely to be associated with a structural lesion than symptoms always felt on the same side.

Migraine tends to follow the same pattern of symptoms from attack to attack, the attacks occurring 'episodically' with no symptoms in between times. A tumour tends to be associated with a progression of symptoms over a relatively short period, the symptoms getting worse with time.

Are there any sources of information that I could give to my son's school so that they can understand a bit more about migraine?

The headache charities are your best source of information. The Migraine Action Association, The Migraine Trust and OUCH UK all have excellent websites and a variety of information leaflets suitable for headache sufferers. See Appendix 1 for their contact details.

NON-DRUG-TREATMENT APPROACHES

Our GP says that my daughter's headaches might be caused by stress. Can children really get stressed?

Anyone can get or feel stressed, and children are no exception. The causes of stress can be different in children, potentially more complex and sometimes difficult to identify or recognise. Life can affect different people in different ways. The effect or impact of life events should never be ignored or underestimated.

Finding out what might be causing stress is often quite difficult and challenging. The only way is to ask around, seeing what friends and family members think or feel about what is going on. Worry about exams, being bullied at school, getting homework finished on time or even the illness of friends or family members may all cause problems that are not readily identified by you or your child. We all react and cope differently to life events. We all cope with and talk about our feelings in different ways and sometimes not at all.

My daughter is keen to go to drama class and chess club. Do you think kids can do too many things after school?

Getting the balance right between things we want to do, need to do and have to do is always difficult. Homework and chores have to be done, eating and sleeping need to be done, after-school clubs and hobbies are things we want to do. Doing too much of everything is not a good idea and may cause stress but doing enough of the good things helps relieve stress.

I am always reluctant to be dogmatic but if she is getting a lot of headaches already, she will need to reflect on how full her days are. It is all about balance. By all means let her try to go to drama and chess club but remember there will still be homework and chores to do.

> *My son, who is at primary school, often gets his migraines in the afternoon. I am not convinced he eats his lunch. Could that be a trigger?*

Yes, it could. If he skips, misses or delays lunch, this may drop his migraine threshold and increase the chance of a migraine developing later in the afternoon. It might be worth having a chat to the staff at the school to see whether he is eating his lunch. If he isn't, you will need to try to find out why. Children can be notoriously faddy and difficult when it comes to food these days. It may be that he will do better with a packed lunch, with a mix of healthy options and the occasional treat.

> *How hard should I try to get my daughter to have breakfast every morning? Is it really worth the effort?*

Changing patterns of behaviour is always challenging but often worth the effort! Eating regularly and drinking enough of the right sort of fluids are important. Breakfast is often referred to as the most important meal of the day because it ends the overnight fast, and the right sort of breakfast will set her up for the morning. It is all about keeping her migraine threshold as high as possible. The higher the threshold, the less likely that a migraine attack will happen.

For more information on the migraine threshold, have a look at Chapter 7.

The specialist nurse has said that if my son stops drinking so much cola he will get fewer headaches. Will it make that much difference?

Cola contains caffeine and sugar or artificial sweeteners. Caffeine can cause headache in its own right, as can artificial sweeteners. Drinking lots of fizzy drinks, especially if they are his sole source of fluid, means that he is less likely to drink enough water and so he could become dehydrated to some degree. Dehydration has the potential to lower his migraine threshold, so drinking plenty of water but little or no cola can raise his headache threshold and make it less likely that he'll have an attack.

How do I get my son to stop drinking fizzy drinks and have water instead?

Your son will have to want to do that for himself. Motivation and ownership of an idea are the best way to encourage the change to happen. Your son must decide for himself that he needs to do whatever it takes to reduce the number of headaches he gets. You can, of course, support him in that process. Only if he makes that decision for himself, though, will he be able to find the motivation to make the change from fizzy drinks to water.

The nurse has said breakfast, lunch and dinner every day. That's easy enough to say but how do you cut down on the junk food?

Changing diet and lifestyle is all about desire and motivation with a hefty dose of insight. Recognising and accepting that avoiding junk food will make your headaches better is the first step to initiating change. Change comes from within and it is never easy to seem to be different. Peer pressure is a powerful force but if the desire for fewer headaches is strong enough, diet changes do happen. Once an improvement occurs, the change becomes the norm and accepted. Improvement will also encourage further changes in behaviour.

*My daughter has a part-time job after school, which means
that she is up quite late sometimes doing her homework. Will
all those late nights mean more migraines?*

Too little sleep, as well as too much sleep, can lead to more
migraines. Late nights along with early mornings can also lead
to more migraines. A regular sleep pattern is the ideal, and a change
in sleep patterns – for whatever reason – can cause a shift in the
migraine threshold. Regular food and fluid intake may help but won't
completely prevent this, and anything that causes a fall in the
migraine threshold has the potential to lead to more migraines.

*Exams are coming up and I'm wondering what I can do to
help my daughter get through without getting any
migraines. Have you any suggestions?*

Exams are a stressful time and there are a variety of approaches
that may work for her. Stress in this situation can be both good
and bad. It is about finding ways to spread the stress as much as possible, or use the stress in a positive and constructive way.

Try to plan regular breaks into the day and the revision. Encourage regular fluid intake and healthy snacks with regular meal breaks.
Think about the range of potential triggers that come into play to
push her migraine threshold down, and control the ones that can be
modified so that the rest become less of an issue. Everyone is different
and different triggers have differing effects at different times.

*My son seems to spend most of his spare time in front of our
PC playing games. Can computer games cause migraines?*

Flickering lights can cause migraines and playing computer games
in a dark room may trigger a migraine attack. Any computer
screen, if used for significant periods in poor lighting conditions,
could push the migraine threshold down and lead to a higher probability of a migraine developing. Posture may also be a factor in

triggering headache symptoms in this situation (see also the next answer).

Should I be discouraging my kids from playing computer games?

This is a difficult one, as things forbidden will often become much more desirable! A little bit of the things we enjoy doing is good for us, but too much of some things may not be quite such a good idea.

As well as the lighting factor (see the previous answer), posture can have an effect in generating headache symptoms. So spending too much time crouched over a computer game could lead to headache symptoms. If there seems to be a direct cause and effect in any of your children, playing fewer computer games may be the answer. Triggers are rarely relevant in total isolation so think about other factors that may come into play at the same time, as these may need to be reviewed or modified as well.

It is always difficult to know the best way to tackle things. All things in moderation is usually a sensible starting point. Banning something is rarely helpful, but restricting the amount of time spent is a reasonable compromise; also, not playing games in the 30 minutes before bedtime might help.

ACUTE DRUG TREATMENTS

What should I use for my daughter's migraine attacks?

It depends on what sort of migraine and what symptoms she gets. If she has aura, taking something such as ibuprofen as soon as the aura starts is a good option. Even if she does not feel nauseated, taking something to encourage the stomach to empty will tend to make the ibuprofen work faster.

If she does not get aura but her attack starts with a headache, the same mix should work well if it is taken early enough.

Should I try ibuprofen or paracetamol to ease the migraine headache my daughter gets?

Either has the potential to work, provided a high enough dose is taken and it is taken early enough. Migraine is an inflammatory process, so ibuprofen should work better than paracetamol. Taking both together may work better than either one alone. Everyone is different, and the best treatment is the one that works best for your daughter – and you won't know which until she tries them both.

My son gets quite bad nausea and vomiting. What can he try to help relieve these symptoms?

The best option is what is referred to as a gastric-emptying anti-emetic – it helps the stomach to empty and should reduce the chance of vomiting. There are two drugs that can be used but domperidone is the one preferred in children. The dose is calculated on the basis of body weight and can be given as a 'suspension' (a liquid) as well as a tablet.

The alternative is metoclopramide, but this is best avoided if your son is under the age of 20 years unless no other option is effective. It can be given in the form of tablets, suspension or injection and, as with domperidone, the dose is calculated according to his body weight.

I would describe my son as being large for his age. Is there a right or wrong dose of ibuprofen to treat his migraine?

The right dose of ibuprofen is the one that works and relieves the headache quickly and completely. There are, of course, dosage guidelines for children in different age groups:

- in 1- to 2-year-olds: 50 mg, three or four times a day
- in 3- to 7-year-olds: 100 mg, three or four times a day
- in 8- to 12-year-olds: 200 mg, three or four times a day

If he is large for his age, I would be inclined to calculate the dose on the basis of his body weight – if you know how much he weighs. The dose is 20–30 mg per kg, split into three or four doses in the day.

Remember that you can use ibuprofen in children under the age of 16, but not aspirin. If ibuprofen does not work, try paracetamol or go back to your GP for more advice.

I have found that my daughter's headache gets better with the first dose of ibuprofen but always comes back. Can I repeat the dose?

Yes, you can. She can take a dose every four to six hours, depending on how much she takes each time. The first dose should be the highest, and each subsequent dose could be slightly lower. The total dose that can be taken over any 24-hour period depends on her age and weight, and this total dose can help you calculate the best dose mix (see the previous answer).

I use paracetamol for my child's headache – is there a right dose? Can I give her too much?

As with ibuprofen you need to use the right dose of paracetamol soon enough in the headache phase of a migraine attack. The correct dose is decided on the basis of age, or body weight if under the age of 3 months, taking no more than four doses in each 24-hour period:

- 3 months to 1 year: 60 to 120 mg every 4 to 6 hours
- 1 to 5 years: 120 to 250 mg every 4 to 6 hours
- 6 to 12 years: 250 to 500 mg every 4 to 6 hours

If the child is under 3 months, the dose is calculated using the formula of 10 mg per kg body weight.

How can I tell that my son has the best treatment for his migraine?

That rather depends on how you define 'best treatment'. The 'best' is usually the one that works the quickest, takes the headache away completely, does not allow the headache to come back during the next 24 to 48 hours and causes few or no side effects.

There is no 'best' option to fulfil all these parameters but a suitable compromise should exist if you seek it out. Different people respond to different drugs and drug combinations and the best is the one that gives your son the best compromise.

My son's treatment seems to work better at the weekend, rather than if an attack occurs at school. Why is that?

This is a difficult question to answer absolutely but treating migraine effectively is all about getting the medication on board quickly. It is generally felt that it may be easier to get treatment on board quickly at home than at school. Access in a school environment may be delayed by needing to get at the medication and also getting water with which to take it. It may also be harder at school to find a quiet place for a short period to allow the medication to take hold.

Why do the pills seem to work better for some attacks rather than others?

Timing is everything when it comes to taking treatment for migraine. 'If I take my tablets quickly enough' is a frequently heard phrase. The earlier pills are taken, the more effective they are in treating the attack. Early treatment tends to get rid of the headache more quickly and means it is less likely to recur in the next 24 to 48 hours.

There are other factors that come into play, and they tend to vary from person to person. The relevant factors may well reflect where the person's migraine threshold is at the time that the attack is triggered.

Another difficulty with youngsters is that the attack may be much shorter than is seen in adults, so the criteria used to assess the response may well not be valid or relevant. If the attack is shorter on occasion, the perception is that the treatment worked better, whereas the attack was settling anyway, regardless of the treatment.

Are there any right or wrong tablets for my son to take for his migraine?

The 'right' tablet is the one that works well in relieving all the symptoms of the migraine attack and stops it from coming back. The 'wrong' tablet is the one that does not relieve the symptoms of the attack or causes unacceptable side effects. Trial and error will discover the ones that help and the ones that don't.

My GP has said that triptans are not licensed for use in children. What does that mean?

Drugs have to go through a formal approval process before they can be prescribed to treat specified conditions. This occurs after their effectiveness and safety have been assessed in drug trials. The process looks at what conditions a drug can be used to treat and for what age groups it can be prescribed.

Drugs can also be prescribed in an 'unlicensed' way, or 'off licence'. This means that experience and common usage have led to a drug being used for other conditions or age groups. Triptans were originally tested only with adults, and are used safely and effectively by them. Recently, however, two triptans have been licensed for use in 12- to 18-year-olds and this would tend to suggest that all of them can probably be used safely in this age group.

How can I decide which triptan to give to my daughter when only two of them are licensed for children?

The triptan to use is the one that works the best. Sumatriptan adolescent nasal spray and zolmitriptan are currently licensed for use in 12- to 18-year-olds, so try those first. If they do not work as well as expected or hoped for, try the others in turn. You will then find one that works in the way you are looking for.

Is it safe to use something that is not licensed?

Using drugs that are not licensed is possible, and in fact may not be that uncommon. It will depend on what aspect of the licence is actually being 'ignored'. With triptans, using a drug 'off licence' usually relates to the age of the person taking the drug. This is the only area where it is reasonable to consider using a triptan in someone under the age of 12 for sumatriptan adolescent nasal spray and zolmitriptan, and under the age of 18 for the other triptans.

It is felt that these rules of age can be broken, provided that the responsible adult, be this a parent or guardian, gives informed consent. There is a need to balance the theoretical risk of using a triptan in these age groups against the benefit in terms of improved quality of life and reduced time off school or work.

How old do you have to be to take triptans?

Age is a relative thing but according to the licence you should be over the age of 12 to take sumatriptan adolescent nasal spray and zolmitriptan, and over the age of 18 for the other triptans.

I take sumatriptan nasal spray and I noticed that the strength is 20 mg but the nasal spray my teenage daughter has been given is only 10 mg. Will hers work as well?

The form of sumatriptan licensed for teens is the 'adolescent nasal spray', which is a dose of 10 mg, whereas the adult dose for the nasal spray is 20 mg. The research evidence suggests it should work as well. If you and your daughter feel that it does not offer the necessary benefit, it is reasonable to ask her doctor if she can try the adult version to see if it is any better.

I use zolmitriptan for my migraines. Why can't my kids use the same if they get migraine?

They can now, if they are 12 or over, because zolmitriptan is one of the two triptans that have been licensed for use between the ages of 12 and 18. Your GP will probably want to check this out, and can do so by looking it up in a reference book known as the *BNF*. The *BNF* is the *British National Formulary*, which lists all the drugs available in the UK to treat any condition.

If sumatriptan adolescent nasal spray and zolmitriptan don't work for my daughter, and they are the only triptans that are licensed for adolescents, can we try one of the other triptans?

Yes, you could but you need to talk to your GP or specialist so that you can discuss the alternatives available and choose which one your daughter wants to try next. They are all worth trying but she will need to treat three consecutive attacks with any given triptan to assess how effective each one is.

It is about informed decision-making and making you, as the parent or guardian, aware of the relevant safety issues and concerns.

My GP has given me lots of information about sumatriptan and zolmitriptan. What other triptans are there?

There are seven different triptans in all, the other five being almotriptan, eletriptan, frovatriptan, naratriptan and rizatriptan; they come in a variety of forms: tablets, wafers or 'melts', nasal sprays and injections. There are pros and cons to each and they each work differently in different people. Trial and error is the only way to find out which one works for your child.

If the triptan eases the headache but doesn't take it away, what else can my daughter try to get rid of her migraine?

She could try the same triptan at a higher dose, if one is available, or a different triptan. All triptans react differently in different people, so all are worth trying to find which works best.

If the various triptan options do not work on their own, it is worth your daughter trying taking an anti-inflammatory such as ibuprofen or a simple painkiller such as paracetamol at the same time as the triptan.

It may be that taking an anti-nausea drug such as domperidone (in preference to metoclopramide) may make the triptan more effective. If this is not enough, a mix of triptan, ibuprofen and domperidone may be needed. It is all about looking at the full range of options out there and ringing the changes until you find what works. Your GP, paediatrician or specialist nurse will be able to provide the necessary advice, information and support needed.

For more information about acute treatment options, look at Chapter 11.

If there are seven triptans, is any one better than the others?

Not really – they all have the ability to work well if taken at the right time at the right dose. Different drugs are 'best' in different people, and what is best for one person may not be best for another.

The choice is complex and based on a variety of factors, including speed of onset (how quickly the treatment works), sustained pain-free response (the headache going away and staying away) and low side effects (not making you feel any worse than you do already).

PREVENTATIVE TREATMENT

When is it time to think about preventative treatment for my son rather than acute treatment?

Preventative treatment is not a substitute for acute treatment because it will not stop all attacks happening. Deciding that prevention is a good idea and finding the motivation to take a tablet every day needs careful thought, as all drugs are potentially associated with side effects and although reducing the total number of headache days will not stop them all.

The point at which preventative medications are tried usually depends on the total number of headache days experienced in each month, balanced against the effectiveness of acute treatments and concerns about the overuse of medications with continued usage. Deciding when preventative treatment is the right thing to do is about balancing a series of factors until a point or 'threshold' is reached; that threshold is different for everyone, adult or child, when it is decided that taking a tablet every day is worth it.

What drugs can be used to prevent migraine in children?

The same drugs used to treat adult migraine can be used in children, the dose depending on the child's weight and age. Drugs include beta-blockers, anti-epileptic drugs, tricyclic antidepressants and pizotifen. All have been shown, in a range of trials, to have some effect in reducing the frequency of migraine attacks.

Is there a preventative drug that works best in children?

The best drug is the one that stops the most number of headache days and causes the least side effects. As with adults, any one child will react differently to each of the drugs available. There is a case to be made to try different drugs in the same class or group, as the effect may vary significantly from one to the next. A drug has to be taken for long enough at the right dose to have its effect.

I am not too sure I want my child to take a tablet every day to stop migraines. Do preventative drugs stop all migraine attacks?

No, they don't. Preventative drugs will only reduce the number of headache days by up to 50% in up to 50% of people. Taking a tablet every day can be a chore and nobody wants to take a tablet every day without good reason. However, the advantages will outweigh the disadvantages if drugs are used for a limited period to break the cycle of frequent headache and return to an infrequent pattern of migraine attacks.

How can I know that my daughter is taking the right dose of the drug?

To minimise the risk of side effects I would suggest starting her at a low dose and then slowly increasing it to an initial 'target dose'. This target dose tends to be the lowest dose at which that drug can be expected to have an effect.

The right dose is the one that reduces the total number of headache days by at least 50%. The number of headache days at each dosing phase needs to be monitored before a further dose increase is considered, assuming that side effects are not a problem. The doctor will review your daughter's response to the drug at three-monthly intervals.

If we decide that my son should take a preventative drug, how long will he need to take it?

He needs to take it for long enough to produce an effect: this is assessed by using diary cards (see Chapter 12) and counting the total number of headache days. Preventative drugs should not be taken permanently but for long enough to break the current cycle of attacks. There is rarely a need to take the drugs for more than six to twelve months.

Assuming that the preventative drugs work for my daughter, what is the best way to stop taking them?

Slowly! A gradual stepped reduction over a few weeks is the safest way to prevent a 'rebound' effect. During this step-down phase it is wise to pay particular attention to diet and lifestyle factors to support the process and keep the migraine threshold as high as possible.

15 | Women, hormones and headaches

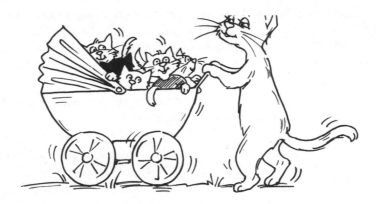

MENSTRUAL MIGRAINE AND MENSTRUALLY ASSOCIATED MIGRAINE

The nurse keeps talking about my menstrual cycle.
What is my menstrual cycle?

A menstrual cycle is the length of time between the first day of one period and the first day of the next period. It can vary by up to seven days, but is usually fairly regular within a day or two. A simple diary recording exactly when you have your period allows you to calculate the length of your menstrual cycle.If you look at the diary shown in Figure 15.1, recorded in the months of March, April and

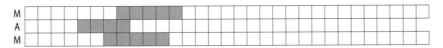

Figure 15.1 A simple diary recording when the period occurred.

May, you can see that the cycle from March to April is 29 days. You can work this out by counting the number of days from the first day of the period on 8 March, to the first day of your period on 5 April. If you count the days in the same way the April to May cycle is 32 days.

My cousin tells me that she has menstrual migraine and she reckons that I have it, too. What exactly is it?

Menstrual migraine, which affects about 10% of women, has a very precise definition. The attack must start no more than two days before the first day of your period and two days after the first day of your period, inclusive, and you cannot have attacks at any other time in your cycle. This must occur and be recorded in two out of three cycles.

If you record a period diary as shown in Figure 15.1, and then mark in the days that you have headache, you and your doctor can see if there is an association between your headaches and your periods.

In the diary shown in Figure 15.2, the areas marked 'H' denote headache days, and as you can see there are no headaches at other times of the cycle. This is menstrual migraine.

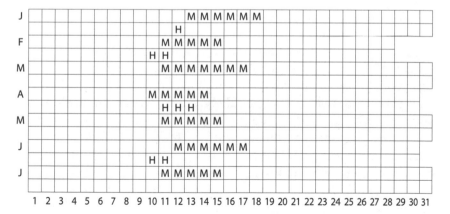

Figure 15.2 Diary noting menstrual period (M) and headache days (H).

I think my migraines are something to do with my periods but how can I prove it?

The best way to prove it is to keep a diary that shows when your period is and when your migraine is. It is a good idea to keep the diary for at least six months, as you may not get a migraine with every period. If you don't record things for long enough, the link may well be missed.

The diary card in Figure 15.3 shows that one attack (in March) may be menstrual migraine but the vast majority of headaches fall outside the definition of menstrual migraine. It is important to remember that some headaches may be migraine but some may be a tension-type headache; you need to understand more about associated symptoms in order to make this distinction.

M						M	M	M	M	M																			
		H				H	H						H			H	H	H					H				
A																													
M	H	H	H					H	H			H						H			H	H					
M						M	M	M	M	M																		
		H				H	H	H							H				H	H							

Figure 15.3 Diary card recording menstrual periods (M) and headache days (H).

Why do I get attacks around the time of my period?

Migraine can occur at any time and may be associated with your period just by chance. Migraine attacks happen when your threshold is low. A variety of factors have the ability to push down your threshold. One of these could be falling oestrogen levels along with dehydration and fluctuating blood sugar levels.

Around the time of your period you tend to get food cravings, often for sweet things. If you reach for the cakes, sweets and biscuits, this tends to produce peaks and troughs in your sugar levels.

It is easy to get stressed and bad tempered around the time of your period. This may lead you to skipping or delaying meals or to having unsettled sleep, all of which could push your migraine threshold down.

***My migraines tend to occur around my period. Is there
anything I can do to stop them happening?***

It rather depends on how you want to tackle it. The first step –
which doesn't involve taking tablets – is to think about diet and
lifestyle changes. Try to keep your blood sugar levels as stable as
possible with low glycaemic index (low GI) foods, eat regularly and
drink plenty of water. Try to keep your caffeine intake – tea, coffee
and colas – low, too.

For more information about diet and lifestyle, look in Chapter 7.

***The nurse at the clinic says I don't have menstrual migraine.
I can get attacks at any time but I always get an attack when
I start my period. If it's not menstrual migraine, what is it?***

It sounds as if you have *menstrually associated migraine*. This term
allows for the attack of true menstrual migraine to be
accompanied by attacks at other times in the cycle as well as at the
start of your period.

As you can see from the diary shown in Figure 15.4, the severe
headaches are almost certainly migraine and the moderate headaches are probably migraine, but the mild headaches are probably

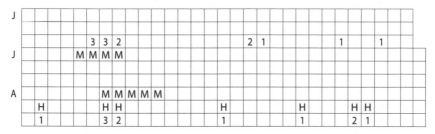

Figure 15.4 Recording headache days (H) and their severity,
and menstrual periods (M).
1 = mild headache, not likely to be migraine; 2 = moderate headache,
possibly migraine; 3 = severe headache, probably migraine

not. The episode of headache at the start of the August period is a severe headache that is probably migraine, but the headaches during the rest of the cycle are mild. The attack before the June period is associated with the period, but there are other episodes of moderate headache (which may be migraine) in that cycle, making the diagnosis menstrually associated migraine rather than menstrual migraine.

I know that I have menstrual migraine. It has been suggested that using hormones might help. How is this?

The hormone concerned is oestrogen rather than progestogen, both being female sex hormones. Research has suggested that it is the size and speed of the fall of oestrogen levels that occurs at the start of the period that have the potential to trigger a migraine.

Hormone treatments are thought to help by slowing down the speed of the fall of oestrogen and thereby reducing the chance of a migraine attack being triggered. The important thing is to get the timing right, and that means starting the oestrogen two days before you expect the attack to happen and using it for seven days. The oestrogen is most effective in the form of a patch or gel, because this delivers steady and even levels of hormone into the bloodstream. The main drawback with this approach is that your periods must be regular: you have to be able to predict when the period will start so that you can begin the treatment two days before.

M						M	M	M	M	M																																	
					H	H																																				
				O	O	O	O	O	O	O																																
J						M	M	M	M	M																																
			H	H	H																																						
	O	O	O	O	O	O	O																																O	O		
J				M	M	M	M	M																																		
			H	H	H																																						
	O	O	O	O	O																																						

Figure 15.5 Diary recording menstrual period (M), migraine days (H) and days when oestrogen was used (O).

As you can see from the diary shown in Figure 15.5, each cycle is of 29 days. The migraine attack starts on a different day in each cycle, so you will need to start your oestrogen four days before the start of your period to anticipate the onset of your migraine. As you can appreciate, your periods really do need to be regular to be able to use this approach.

I am happy to try oestrogen to stop my menstrual attacks happening but why do I have to use a patch rather than a tablet?

Hormone-dependent attacks are triggered by fluctuating oestrogen levels and the degree and rate of change are the factors that need to be modified to prevent attacks from happening. A patch allows a steady, even level of hormone to develop in the bloodstream. A tablet, however, has to go through the stomach and intestine to be absorbed, and many factors may affect how well it is absorbed. Varying rates of absorption of oestrogen lead to fluctuations in hormone levels that are less than ideal for the task.

I have tried several different patches but am sensitive to the adhesive. Using the oestrogen seems to work really well, though, so is there anything else I can try?

One trick, if you have not tried it yet, is to wave the patch in the air before applying it. Sometimes it is the alcohol that causes a reaction rather than the adhesive itself. If that does not work, you could try an oestrogen gel instead. The gel gives a steady level of oestrogen in the same way the patch does.

My GP has suggested that I take naproxen regularly to stop my menstrual attack happening. Is it really going to work?

Naproxen is a non-steroidal anti-inflammatory drug (NSAID) that works by targeting a particular chemical called *prostaglandin*.

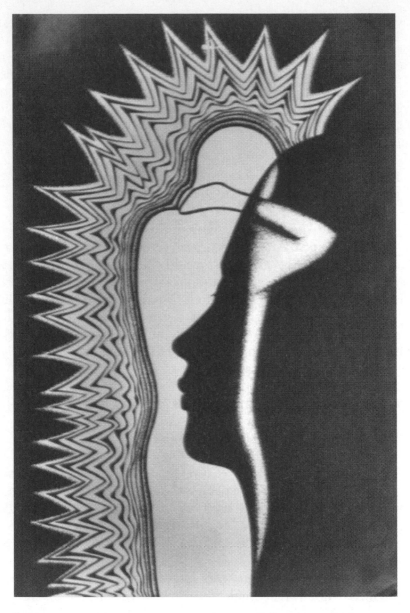

Plate 2 From the Migraine Art collection, reproduced by kind permission of the Migraine Action Association and Boehringer Ingelheim

						M	M	M	M	M																			
					H	H																							
			N	N	N	N	N	N	N																				
					M	M	M	M																					
		H	H	H																									
N	N	N	N	N	N	N																				N	N		
		M	M	M	M																								
	H	H	H																										
N	N	N	N	N	N	N																							

Figure 15.6 Diary recording menstrual period (M), migraine days (H) and days when naproxen was used (N).

Prostaglandin levels are known to rise during a period and have been shown to trigger a migraine-like headache. Anything that can stop the rise in prostaglandin levels should reduce the chance of a migraine being triggered (see Figure 15.6).

If you get painful periods, you could continue to take the naproxen to the end of your period to relieve these symptoms.

If you start the naproxen two days before you expect the migraine to happen and take it for seven days, there is a fair chance that the attack will not be triggered. You have to be able to predict exactly when your period is going to be for this option to be viable.

I have painful periods and always get a migraine on the first or second day of my period. My GP has suggested I take a non-steroidal anti-inflammatory. Why will this help me?

Prostaglandins are chemicals released by the lining of the womb, causing the pain of painful periods. They are also associated with the triggering of migraine attacks. Using a non-steroidal anti-inflammatory drug (NSAID) such as naproxen or ibuprofen can suppress the level of prostaglandins in the blood and thus reduce the chance of a migraine happening as well as helping the pain of your period.

Are all non-steroidal anti-inflammatories the same? I know the names are different but if one doesn't work, is it worth trying another?

Each NSAID does seem to work differently in different people at different times. If one doesn't seem to work for you, it is certainly worth trying a different one. There can also be a 'dose response' aspect as well, so, if the lower dose does not work, try a higher one. Remember that the drug has to be taken regularly to be effective in preventing an attack from developing.

My menstrual attacks are really hard to treat. What is the best way of getting rid of the migraine?

It is not clear why menstrual attacks are often difficult to treat. If you usually use a triptan to treat your migraine, you need to think about using the top dose of whichever one you take. For example:

- *Sumatriptan*: try 100 mg instead of 50 mg, or the nasal spray instead of the tablets.

- *Zolmitriptan*: try the 5 mg dose rather than 2.5 mg, or the nasal spray instead of tablets.

- *Eletriptan*: think about using 80 mg rather than 40 mg or 20 mg.

If the triptan you use has only a single dose option or if the maximum dose doesn't allow you to be headache-free or does not prevent headache recurrence, think about using a mix of drugs to do the job. This may mean using a triptan and an NSAID along with an anti-nausea drug such as domperidone or metoclopramide. You need to use what is called a pro-kinetic anti-nausea drug to promote emptying of the stomach and thus help all the drugs be absorbed.

If this mix gets rid of the headache but it tends to recur, you may have to repeat the dose of the NSAID through the course of the next 24 to 36 hours to be sure of hitting the attack on its head.

Zolmitriptan works quite well for most of my attacks but my menstrual attacks just don't seem to settle as well. Any suggestions?

I suggest that you try zolmitriptan, either the 5 mg Rapimelt, or two 2.5 mg tablets or the nasal spray. If that is not enough, add in naproxen or ibuprofen. Naproxen should be used in a dose of 500 mg, and you can repeat the dose in about 12 hours. Ibuprofen can be used in a dose of 400 mg, 600 mg or even 800 mg. The dose can be repeated in six to eight hours but you must not take more than 2,400 mg in any 24-hour period.

I have found that naproxen seems to work better than ibuprofen for my menstrual attacks. Why is this?

Different drugs do work differently in different people, and it may be that naproxen is the one that suits you. There is a suggestion that naproxen may target just the right prostaglandin that is released during your period and is involved in triggering migraine.

I want to try to prevent some of my migraines. Some are around my period and some occur at any time. What can I do?

There are lots of options and any one of them might help you. It may be that you need to think about all the options, but try each one alone before trying different combinations until you find what works for you.

Diet and lifestyle changes are always a good start. Eating regularly, drinking lots of water, trying low glycaemic index (GI) foods and having regular breaks to de-stress through the day can all help.

If making these changes helps a little but you want to try something else, you need to decide whether you want to try a preventative drug. This means taking something every day to try to reduce the number of headache days you get throughout the month. Alternatively, you might want to try a targeted option – taking the preventative drug just prior to your menstrual attack – but it won't help attacks at other times of the cycle.

The choices are yours and yours alone but your GP, specialist or specialist nurse are there to support you through the decision-making.

I don't really want to take a tablet every day to stop my migraines. Is there anything else I can do?

If you do not want to take preventative drugs, you will need to focus on diet and lifestyle changes or consider 'targeted' treatment focused on your menstrual attacks. If neither of these has enough of an effect, though, you will need to think about preventative drugs, but to work they will have to be taken every day.

If you have attacks throughout your cycle, intermittent treatment around your period isn't going to have a significant impact on the total number of headache days. It is a trade-off because, if your menstrual attacks are stopped and these are hardest to treat, stopping them may be the best option for you.

PREGNANCY

I'm expecting our first baby. Am I more or less likely to get migraine while I am pregnant?

If you get menstrual migraine, there is a 60–70% chance that you will have few or no migraines while pregnant. This is even more likely if you normally get migraine without aura.

Up to 25% of women get no change in migraine frequency while they are pregnant but, unfortunately, 4–8% find that their attacks get worse. They are more likely to get worse if you normally get migraine with aura.

My sister did not get any migraines while she was pregnant but I do. Why are we different?

It would be fair to say that no one really knows why but it is assumed that it is something to do with the steady level of oestrogen that occurs during pregnancy. Pregnancy is divided into three 'trimesters' and migraine might get worse in the first trimester and then improve in the second and third trimesters.

Your situation is more likely to improve if you have migraine without aura. You are more likely to get migraine with aura for the first time during pregnancy and it is more likely to get worse during pregnancy.

I have always had migraines around the time of my period. Will they get better or worse while I am pregnant?

Migraine around the time of your period, especially if it is true menstrual migraine, is normally migraine without aura. The expectation would be that the migraine will get better, especially in the second and third trimesters.

Are there any headaches that occur during pregnancy that I should be worried about?

A serious (or 'sinister') headache can occur at any time, not just during pregnancy. The main concern in pregnancy is a headache that is associated with pre-eclampsia or eclampsia.

Pre-eclampsia is a condition that can occur at any stage in pregnancy and is associated with a rise in blood pressure, swelling of your feet and/or fingers and protein in your urine.

Eclampsia is the next step and much more serious. The headache will often become much more severe, the blood pressure higher and may be associated with changes in the level of consciousness and, occasionally, fits.

If you are worried about your headaches, talk to your GP or midwife about them.

I am six months pregnant and occasionally get blurred vision with a bad headache. Should I go and see my GP or midwife?

Any change in your vision should not really be ignored. It could be related to your blood pressure or possibly a rise in the pressure in your eye. The latter, called *glaucoma*, can be associated with eye pain or headache.

Blurring of your vision is not usually a feature of migraine aura unless it is what is referred to as stereotypical – meaning that the pattern is consistent and blurring is more of a visual distortion rather than just a slight loss of focus.

If you get new symptoms or a change in symptoms, it is always important to seek advice. If you don't want to bother your GP in the first instance, you could see your optometrist and, if this assessment seems normal, see your GP or midwife.

I am a little concerned as I got these horrible flashing lights in the middle of my vision when I was pregnant. I never got a headache to follow. What was this all about?

Migraine with aura can occur for the first time in pregnancy, although it is not clear why. The flashing lights might have been a migraine aura. As is the case when you are not pregnant, it is possible to get an aura but not have a headache follow it.

My mother got her first migraine when she was pregnant with me. My sister and aunt get migraine, but I have never had one. I have just got pregnant and wonder what are my chances of getting a migraine while pregnant?

The optimistic view would be low, the pessimistic view would be high and the realistic view is 'who knows'. If you have a family history of migraine, you have an above average chance of developing migraine at some time. Migraine can develop at any time and pregnancy is as good a time as any.

I have never had migraine before but I developed migraine with aura during the early part of my pregnancy. Should I be concerned, and will I always get them now?

Not easy questions to answer! If you have a family history of migraine, you could develop migraine at any time, and migraine with aura is more likely to occur for the first time during pregnancy. It is important that you ask your doctor for a full assessment in order to confirm that there are no symptoms, or 'red flags', to cause concern, and make sure that on examination there are no abnormalities to be found to suggest a structural cause. (For more information about 'red flags', see Chapter 5.)

Aura tends to follow a typical pattern and, provided that what you experience fits with what is regarded as normal, there is little cause for concern. If the aura symptoms are not typical, your GP might refer you to a neurologist, to exclude any possible 'sinister' cause, especially when they occur for the first time.

I'm afraid it is impossible to say whether your migraine will continue after the baby is born. Only time will tell.

My migraines have settled while I have been pregnant but what's going to happen when my baby arrives?

If you are lucky, you may not get a 'rebound' effect immediately after the baby arrives. Unfortunately, the evidence suggests that as many as 40% of women who have migraine get their migraines back after the baby is born.

What can I take to treat my migraine while I am pregnant?

Hopefully, you won't get many migraines while you are pregnant, because your options are limited in real terms to paracetamol. If you get significant symptoms and their severity justifies using other drugs to aid the nausea and vomiting, you could take an anti-nausea drug, but this may be discouraged in the way that the use of any drug during pregnancy is discouraged. See the next few answers for more information.

Some people have found that ginger in its various forms – biscuits, tea, cordial – may help some of your nausea symptoms.

> *I have been told that all I can take for my migraine while I am pregnant is paracetamol. Why can't I take anything else?*

As I am sure you know, no drug is encouraged during pregnancy other than iron supplements and folic acid. The reason for this is that at any stage in the pregnancy a drug might have an effect on the growth and development of the baby. Different drugs tend to have different effects and degrees of effects at different stages of the pregnancy.

Over time a database has been built up to try to evaluate exactly what effects drugs have. This information tends to be 'opportunistic' (not the result of scientific research), and often reflects the fact that women have taken drugs in the very early stages before they realised they were pregnant.

Deciding to take anything during pregnancy is about balancing the potential risk of the drug affecting the developing baby and the potential consequence of not managing a problem that needs treating. Discuss the benefits and risks with your doctor or midwife before making a decision.

> *What can I do if my migraine gets worse while I am pregnant?*

Any drug is best avoided in pregnancy. Preventing migraine by following a diet and lifestyle regimen that will keep your threshold as high as possible is a vital first step to staying in control. Making a decision to take drugs is about weighing up the risks and benefits to you and to your baby, which do change in the different stages of pregnancy.

Some drugs that are used to treat migraine are also used for other conditions, and occasionally the potential benefit may well outweigh the theoretical risks of using these drugs in pregnancy.

Talk to your doctor or midwife about lifestyle changes you can make now and what the options might be if your migraines get worse.

How does the specialist decide what I can take to treat my migraine while I am pregnant?

It is never an easy decision to make and tends to depend on the severity of the symptoms you are experiencing and whether the benefit of taking something outweighs the risk.

Some drugs, such as beta-blockers and antidepressants, that can be used to treat migraine, are also used to treat high blood pressure and depression during your pregnancy. These drugs are introduced because not treating the high blood pressure or depression would have a detrimental effect on both mother and baby. Starting these drugs to treat migraine does depend, though, on whether you feel that the possible risk is worth it.

I am taking a preventative drug for my migraine but want to get pregnant. Do I need to stop it?

It is a good idea to stop and see what happens to the frequency of your migraines as a result. The probability is that things will be OK. The advice will always be 'avoid any drug during pregnancy' if at all possible. Some drugs carry a lower risk of harm than others, *but* taking any drug needs careful thought and consideration.

Beta-blockers:

- cause intra-uterine growth retardation (slow the growth of the baby in the womb)

- cause bradycardia (slowing of the heart rate) after birth

- cause hypoglycaemia (very low blood sugar) after birth

Anti-epilepsy drugs (AEDs):

- when used to treat epilepsy the risk of harm outweighs the risk of treatment

- when used to treat epilepsy the risk of harm increases if more than one drug is used at the same time

- there is increased risk of neural tube (spina bifida) and other defects associated with any AED but especially with

  – Epilim (sodium valproate)

  – carbamazepine

  – oxcarbazepine

  – phenytoin

If I stop my preventative drug, will my migraines get worse? If they do get worse, what can I do?

There is no way of knowing if they will get worse but they shouldn't. No preventative drug is taken permanently, so they will have to be stopped some time. The best way to stop it is to reduce the dose slowly, in steps, until you stop taking it altogether. During the phase of 'stepping down' and stopping the drug you need to really focus on the diet and lifestyle areas to keep your migraine threshold as high as you can.

I am planning to breast-feed and wondered what I can take to treat my migraine?

Paracetamol is top of the list. If you need something different, you could try ibuprofen but aspirin and other NSAIDs are to be avoided, as should codeine.

If you need something to help the nausea and/or vomiting, opt for domperidone rather than metoclopramide; you could try prochlorperazine if you cannot tolerate domperidone.

CONTRACEPTION

My sister, who also gets migraine, was told she could not go on the Pill. Why is that?

It rather depends on what sort of migraine she gets. If she gets migraine with aura, current guidelines recommend that she should not go on the combined oral contraceptive pill – that is to say, she can't take a Pill containing oestrogen. However, there is no reason why she can't use the progesterone-only pill, progesterone injection or progesterone-containing coil.

I have been on the Pill for about two years. I got an aura with my last two attacks, and my GP has told me to stop taking the Pill. Why do I have to stop?

It is all to do with risk and your risk of developing a stroke, specifically an *ischaemic stroke*. An ischaemic stroke occurs as a result of a reduction or loss of blood supply to part of the brain.

It is estimated that between 1 and 3 women per 100,000 women under the age of 35 years may experience an ischaemic stroke. On an individual level your chance is very low but there are other risk factors that need to be considered and migraine is one of them. Other factors include smoking, being overweight and taking the combined Pill.

Having migraine increases your chance of having a stroke by three and a half to four times. Migraine with aura carries twice the risk of migraine without aura. If you smoke and have migraine, your risk is increased by ten times. Taking the Pill and smoking increases your risk by 34 times.

As you can see, the risks tend to be cumulative. Although the absolute numbers are quite small, the nature of the cumulative risk cannot really be ignored and the fact that you have developed aura is the decider.

Why has my GP told me that if I want to stay on the Pill I should stop smoking?

If you have migraine without aura and more than one risk factor for stroke, you should stop the Pill – assuming you mean the combined oral contraceptive (COC) pill. Smoking is a potent risk factor, and having migraine and being a smoker and being on the COC pill is not a wise mix. All these, as well as other risk factors such as being overweight or having a high cholesterol, are reasons to think about stopping the Pill.

I know I am overweight but I need reliable contraception. I have been told that, because I smoke, I really should not go on the Pill. Why not?

If you have migraine without aura and want to go on the combined oral contraceptive (COC) pill, you should either lose weight or stop smoking – or, ideally, both. It is about cumulative risk factors and too many risks become a 'no'.

If you feel unable to do either of those things, you need to consider a contraceptive option that does not involve oestrogen. From a hormone point of view, that would be the progesterone-only pill, progesterone injection or coil.

Topiramate works really well as a preventative drug but I'm having problems with using the Depo injection for contraception. Why can't I go back on the Pill?

Topiramate is an anti-epilepsy drug that is known to stimulate or induce liver enzymes to work harder. This means that any drug that is processed by the liver before getting into the circulation is broken down or inactivated more quickly, and so less of the drug is active or 'bioavailable' to do the job it is meant to do.

Any drug taken by mouth has to be processed by the liver and its bioavailability is affected as a result. Going back on the Pill is possible *but* it would be less reliable from a contraceptive point of view, because more of the hormone would be broken down by the liver and less would be available to have its contraceptive effect.

I have been started on topiramate for my migraine. What are my contraceptive options?

Your best options, in terms of effectiveness and reliability, would be progestogen-only injections or the LNG-IUS (levonorgestrel intra-uterine system). The former is given every 10 to 12 weeks and the latter is a coil that is impregnated with progestogen that is slowly released within the womb; once fitted, the coil can stay in place for five years.

I am keen to go back on the Pill despite being on topiramate, as it controls my periods better than the injection. What can I do to make it more reliable as a contraceptive?

You could go back on the Pill but you would have to double up on your contraception in order to increase the contraceptive effect. You could do this by taking a stronger pill – a 50 µg pill, which is no longer available as a standard 'off-the-shelf' prescribable option, so you would have to double up with one that is still available *or* you might opt to use condoms with or without spermicides. You will need to chat to your GP or visit your local family planning clinic for more advice.

I want to stay on the Pill, as it suits me really well. What could I take to reduce the total number of migraine days I get?

You could try valproate, gabapentin or levetiracetam. These are all anti-epilepsy drugs that will not have an effect on the contraceptive reliability of your Pill and have all been shown to have some effect in preventing migraine – they are not liver enzyme 'inducers'.

I am on the Pill, having been using condoms while taking topiramate, which I'll be stopping soon. How long do we need to carry on using condoms?

You should continue to use condoms for four weeks after you have stopped taking topiramate. This allows your liver enzymes to get back to normal so that the Pill can work as effectively as possible, once its bioavailability is back to normal.

DURING AND AFTER THE MENOPAUSE, AND HRT

Everybody says my migraines will get better when I stop having periods. Are they right?

There is a good chance that your migraines will improve once you reach the menopause and have stopped having any periods. Unfortunately, there is also a chance that they will get worse or even stay the same. There is no way of knowing or predicting what will happen.

I am convinced that my migraines have started to get worse now that I am getting some sweats and flushes. Is this because I am becoming menopausal?

Probably, is the simple answer. Sweats and flushes are common in and around the time of the menopause. Menopausal symptoms are caused by fluctuating hormone levels, and it is quite likely that it is these peaks and troughs in oestrogen levels that lower your threshold so that migraine attacks are triggered more easily.

My gynaecologist has suggested that I have a hysterectomy.
I have really bad periods and my migraines are getting
worse. Will the hysterectomy help?

A hysterectomy will definitely help the periods but will probably make the migraines worse. Evidence suggests that a natural menopause reduces the chance of having migraine to about 7% whereas having a 'surgical' menopause leaves you with a 27% chance of getting migraine if you have no premenstrual syndrome (PMS) symptoms. Not the best of odds, I am afraid.

See also the next question and answer.

I used to get bad premenstrual syndrome when I was a
teenager and it is getting bad again. The migraines are
kicking off as well. My periods are irregular and really
heavy. Is hysterectomy the best option?

P remenstrual syndrome (PMS) is not much fun at the best of times and is not easy to treat. It is often associated with migraine-type headaches and migraine can also occur more closely associated with the period. Regulating the period cycle is a good idea, as it may make it easier to control the PMS. Hysterectomy is not the best of options: the evidence suggests that a 'surgical' menopause with a history of PMS gives you a 44% chance of getting migraine afterwards compared with 7% without an operation.

I stopped having periods last year. I have never had an aura
in my life but last month I became aware of short episodes
of flashing lights, just like forked lightning. They last 15 to
20 minutes each time but I don't always get a headache.
Should I be worried?

I t is not uncommon to experience aura in the absence of headache and is a recognised entity. If you have never ever had aura, it is a good idea to see your GP so that a full assessment can be made to rule out any other possible cause for the aura developing. It is a good idea to check your blood pressure, cholesterol and other similar risk factors for stroke. It may even be necessary to have a brain scan to be absolutely certain that the aura is just migrainous. That decision is best made by a specialist.

For information about 'red flag' symptoms, see Chapter 5.

> **My migraines seem to have got worse as my periods have got more irregular. The specialist has suggested I see my GP to discuss HRT but I have read so much about it in magazines that I am not sure what to do. Why is HRT a good idea?**

HRT can help some of the people some of the time. There are, of course, a lot of pros and cons, and the decision-making is nowhere near as easy or straightforward as it used to be. HRT is believed to help by keeping your oestrogen levels as even and steady as possible, because it is thought that it is the peaks and troughs in oestrogen levels that may push down your migraine threshold to a point where triggers are more easily able to generate a migraine attack.

> **I always thought that HRT protected you against stroke, at least that is what my aunt was told when she started HRT ten years ago. My GP has said that it increases the risk of stroke. What has changed?**

Over recent years a lot more research has been completed that has looked at the long-term effects of using HRT. A careful review and analysis of these studies suggests that, on the basis of the best current evidence, the use of HRT increases your chance of ischaemic stroke by 1.29. There is no evidence that it has an effect on haemorrhagic stroke (1.07) or transient ischaemic attack (1.07).

What do these figures mean? If the number is '1', this means that there is no difference. If the number is less than 1, this means that you are less likely to have a problem; if the number is more than 1, you

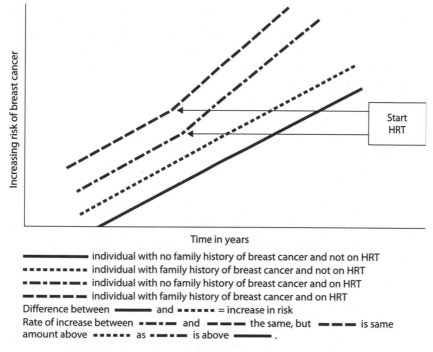

Figure 15.7 Comparative risks of breast cancer with HRT.

are more likely to have a problem. The bigger the number the greater the risk of an event happening.

My mother and her sister both had breast cancer.
My migraines have got much more frequent during the last
few months. I am getting sweats and flushes and my periods
are all over the place. I have been thinking about going on
HRT, but will it make a difference and what are the risks?

If you are getting a lot of menopausal symptoms, tend to get menstrual migraine and want to find a way of regulating your periods, HRT may well help you. If you are under the age of 50, on the basis of current evidence, there is no perceived risk because all you are doing is replacing those hormones that you are not producing consistently.

If you are over the age of 50, the current evidence suggests that you can use HRT for up to five years with no significant increase in risk of developing breast cancer.

What you need to think about is your personal risk of developing breast cancer on the basis of your family history. You have quite a strong family history of breast cancer, which will tend to raise your personal risk, or chance, of developing breast cancer. This risk is higher than in someone with no family history of breast cancer.

There is an increase in risk of developing breast cancer once you have been on HRT for five years or more. Your personal level of risk, and hence your starting point, is higher; going on HRT does not magnify this risk any further, your line just runs along a little higher. See Figure 15.7 for the comparative risks of breast cancer with HRT.

> **I have been thinking about starting HRT to try to help my migraines. My GP has said that I am more likely to get a blood clot in the first year of taking HRT. How likely am I to get a blood clot? Is it worth the risk?**

Your second question is quite difficult to answer because you are the one who should decide whether it is worth the risk. You need to try to assess your personal risk of getting a DVT (deep venous thrombosis – blood clot in the leg).

Age is also a factor: the older you are, the more likely you are to get a DVT. The statistics are given as [number] per 1,000 women in five years. For example:

Age group	Risk without HRT	Risk with HRT
50s	3	7
60s	8	17

There are other times when your risk is increased: when you have been immobile for a prolonged period of time, or anything else that slows your circulation.

I've heard of the coil for contraception. What is a Mirena coil?

A Mirena coil is a specific type of coil that has been impregnated with a particular hormone that is released slowly into the womb. It is also referred to as an LNG-IUS, 'LNG' standing for levonorgestrel and 'IUS' standing for intra-uterine system. Originally developed as a form of contraception, it is now used to treat heavy periods and can also provide the progesterone needed for protection of the womb lining when using oestrogen patches or gel for HRT.

If it is the oestrogen that helps the migraine and I need HRT to help the migraine, why can't I just take oestrogen? That way I won't get periods.

The reason you can't take oestrogen alone, if you have not had a hysterectomy, is that you have to protect the lining of the womb. The lining of the womb – the endometrium – can be over-stimulated when oestrogen is taken on its own and may lead to endometrial cancer.

Five in 1,000 women who are aged between 50 and 64 years of age might expect to develop endometrial cancer if they do not use HRT. Nine in 1,000 women, of the same age, using oestrogen alone for five years might expect to develop endometrial cancer. Obviously, the longer you use oestrogen, the greater the risk. Fifteen in 1,000 women who use oestrogen alone for ten years might expect to develop endometrial cancer.

Using combined HRT is essential, as the numbers then drop dramatically. Fewer than 2 in 1,000 women using combined HRT for ten years might expect to develop endometrial cancer.

> *I had a hysterectomy several years ago because of fibroids
> and am thinking about starting HRT to try to help my
> menopausal symptoms and my migraines. What should
> I use?*

The advantage of having had a hysterectomy is that all you need
to think about is oestrogen. Ideally, you should use a patch or gel.
If you start at a low dose and gradually increase it, you will minimise
the chance of an increase of migraines rather than a hoped-for fall in
the number of attacks.

> *I am using HRT and am trying to decide how long I should
> take it. It has really helped my migraines but I've been
> reading about HRT and breast cancer. How long can I safely
> take it?*

Answering that question is about trying to understand the figures
from research, which looks at population risk, and translating
that into your personal risk. If you are over 50, the longer you take
HRT, the greater your potential personal risk.

Different organisations present the figures in different ways, and
trying to make sense of it all is not easy. If you consider women aged
50 who do not use combined HRT, 32 in every 1,000 would be diagnosed by the age of 65 years.

If you start combined HRT at the age of 50 and take it for five years,
there are 6 extra cases of breast cancer, and if you take it for ten years
there are 19 extra cases. This translates to 38 in every 1,000 who
take combined HRT for five years and 51 in every 1,000 who take
combined HRT for ten years.

Only you can decide how long you can safely take HRT. It depends
on how you weigh up the risks and benefits of taking HRT. This is a
very personal choice and a very individual decision.

I have been on HRT for five years and my migraines have been fantastic. My GP says I have to stop after five years but can I carry on using it?

If you have been on combined HRT for five years, you need to consider the facts and decide what level of risk you are prepared to accept to achieve the benefit you are experiencing. If you feel that the risk of developing breast cancer and the potential increase in risk of stroke are worth it, you can make an informed decision to continue.

If you are taking oestrogen alone and do not need any progesterone for protection of the womb lining, the increase in risk of breast cancer is minimal. There is only one extra case of breast cancer per 1,000 women after five years' use, and a further five cases after ten years.

I have been talking to my GP about HRT after my specialist said I should try it. Tablets, patches or gels: how do I decide?

Patches and gels are going to offer a better option than tablets. It is the peaks and troughs that tend to trigger migraine attacks, and patches and gels will provide a steady blood level.

The advantage of patches, when using a 'matrix' patch, is that you can cut it into quarters and halves and thereby slowly increase the dose of oestrogen. The slower the increase, the easier it is to get control of the migraine without causing a rebound increase in migraine attacks due to too much oestrogen.

I am still getting periods but they are irregular and some of them can be quite heavy. How can I ease my periods and help my migraine?

One option is the low-dose combined Pill, provided you don't smoke and don't get aura. If you get menstrual migraine, you could 'tri-cycle' the Pill, which would reduce the number of periods and the number of migraines. This works because if you take the Pill in the normal way, you get thirteen periods a year. If you tri-cycle the

Pill, take three packs one after the other; then you will get only five periods a year and therefore, potentially, only five migraines.

Another option would be the LNG-IUS (Mirena) coil, which would potentially stop your periods. If this, in itself, is not enough to help the migraines, you might consider top-up oestrogen to stabilise fluctuating hormone levels.

> ***I last had a period two years ago and I am thinking about starting HRT to try to reduce the number of migraines I am getting. I don't want to start periods again, though, so what are my options?***

If it has been that long since you had a period, you could try a continuous combined HRT (CCHRT). This has reasonable chance of giving you bleed-free HRT. You might get some irregular spotting or bleeding but, if CCHRT suits you, you should get few or no periods.

If you do not settle with an off-the-shelf option of CCHRT (one of the standard prescribable options), it is possible to get a little more creative. There are two progestogen products that can be taken on a daily basis and then you can use top-up oestrogen, but start at a low dose and slowly increase it until you get the balance right.

> ***Every time I start HRT, my migraines get worse. Why is this?***

It is probably because you started with too much oestrogen too quickly. The only way to combat this is to start again at a low dose of oestrogen and then slowly increase it. You also need to take progesterone. If you are just starting with menopausal symptoms (being peri-menopausal), it needs to be given cyclically; that is to say, you will need to take the progesterone for a short part of each cycle – giving you a period on a regular basis. If you are two years beyond the menopause and you are using oral progesterone, it should be taken daily. An alternative would be to use the LNG-IUS coil as the progesterone source.

Oestrogen, in this circumstance, is best delivered by a 'matrix' oestrogen patch, which you can cut into quarters and halves. The size of the dose can be manipulated by quartering the patch and increasing the dose by the smallest increment – doing this weekly, fortnightly or monthly. Increasing the dose in this way will allow you to find the amount of oestrogen that will control your migraines and, hopefully, improve any menopausal symptoms you have.

If my migraine gets worse with the tablet HRT, why will patches be better?

The theory is that tablet HRT causes peaks and troughs in oestrogen levels, which might increase the risk of migraines being triggered. Patches will produce a steady level of oestrogen and are therefore less likely to trigger migraines.

My GP has said that too much oestrogen is as much of a problem as too little, so how can I find the right dose and get the balance right?

Finding the right dose and getting the right balance need time and patience if an off-the-shelf formulation does not suit you. Different types of progesterone suit different people, and the dose of oestrogen needs to be just right. This means that you and your doctor need to ring the changes and permutations until you get it right.

16 | Research and the future

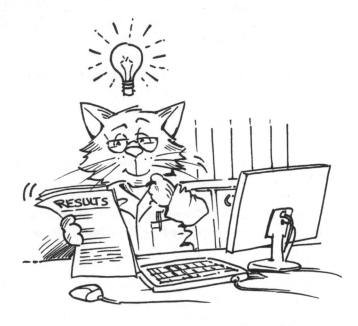

In writing this chapter I have had to reflect on the current state of knowledge and to answer some of my own questions along the way. You need to understand what scientific research is about before you can understand how to interpret the results that make the headlines. You need to be sure that the information presented is not just spin before you can decide that a treatment or intervention is worth the risk and does actually offer any benefit. I hope that what follows answers some of your questions as to what research is all about and what the future might offer the headache sufferer.

The internet has ensured that a vast amount of information is readily accessible. However, you need to be sure that the quality of that information is high and relevant to you. The best place to start is usually the UK-based headache charity websites. They will often have links to other reputable and well-researched websites. Try to stick to

UK-based sites, as some drugs and interventions mentioned on sites in other countries may well not be available in the UK.

RESEARCH: THE WHYS AND WHEREFORES

Why is research important?

There would be no new drugs without research. Research is crucial to our understanding of how the brain works – without that knowledge, scientists and clinicians would not be able to suggest ways of tackling medical conditions and altering or modifying the progress of disease.

Without research we would not have brain scanners, we would not have triptans and we would not know the best and safest ways of repairing holes in the heart or removing brain tumours.

Why is research relevant in migraine?

Research is relevant because without asking questions we cannot understand what is happening, and without knowing what is happening we cannot find ways of changing or modifying it.

In the context of migraine, if scientists had not found out about 5-HT receptors and what they do, we would not have had triptans.

As more is understood about 5-HT receptors, better triptans or other drugs can be developed that work more effectively.

What is 'anecdotal' evidence, and why do we have to prove that something works when people I know tell me it works?

When choosing a holiday or a place to stay, listening to someone else's experience can be helpful in deciding whether you want to go to a particular place or stay in the same hotel. The downside is that if, when you get there, the weather is bad or the hotel is run by different people, your experience might not be as good – so you would never go there again. A few days, weeks or months later, someone else goes there and has a great time – do you go back or not?

That is decision-making based on 'anecdotal' evidence. If you reflect on the example above and transfer that sort of decision-making across to medicine, the issues raised and challenges faced become potentially quite difficult and in some instances even life-threatening.

Any decision you make needs to be sound, safe and cause no harm, hence the need for research and, above all, good research.

What is good research?

Good research is about making sure you ask the right question, in the right way, and set about answering that question using all the right resources, in the right way.

In the context of migraine and triptans you need to evaluate a series of features and factors. To name just a few:

- Is this drug safe?
  - in everyone?
  - in the young?
  - in the elderly?
  - in those who are pregnant?
- Does the drug work?
- Is there a right dose or an optimal dose?
  - does the maximum dose cause too many side effects?
  - does the dose vary in different age groups?
- Is the patient headache-free?
  - in one hour?
  - in two hours?
  - in four hours?
- Is the headache only eased?

Any piece of research must be able to answer all of these questions and many, many more.

How should good trials be constructed?

A good trial needs a clear starting point, which means asking a clear and precise question or series of questions. In the context of preventative drugs or interventions:

- Will X reduce the total number of headache days?

- Will X reduce the total number of headache days by more than 50%?

- Will X make the headache easier to treat with current acute treatment?

- Does X cause side effects?

- What are those side effects?

- Are those side effects sufficient to cause the patient to stop taking the drug?

- Does X perform better than a placebo?

- Does X perform better than the drug the patient was using before?

- Does X perform better than the 'gold standard' or most commonly used drug for, in this case, migraine prevention?

The patients recruited to the study must have the correct diagnosis; in this case the standard is migraine as defined by the International Headache Society.

There must be enough people recruited to the study to ensure that any statistical analysis will have value.

There should at the very least be a placebo or 'dummy' group, and, if feasible, a comparison with a drug already used to treat the condition. No one, that is to say neither the people who are co-ordinating the study and reviewing the patients in the study nor those involved or participating in the study, should know if they are taking active drug or placebo (this is called 'double blind'). If there is a placebo group, it is always interesting to swap this group over to the active drug and assess their response, and vice versa (referred to as 'cross over').

There has to be a baseline period to collect and collate information, in the form of diary cards, to better understand the group being studied. Patients in the trial must stop all other drugs that may have been used, usually for a minimum of four weeks.

There needs to be a minimum number of headache days and a maximum number of headache days recorded within this baseline period, so that patients meet clear recruitment criteria.

Once the trial drug is started, there must be a clear method of increasing the dose, over fixed time intervals, to monitor how effective it is and any side effects (adverse events). There is often a balance between effectiveness and side effects. There must also be a clear way of recording side effects, and identifying at what dose these develop.

The study drug has to be taken long enough to ensure that the full effect of treatment (e.g. maximal reduction in headache days) is recognised and seen, and a follow-up to assess how long the benefit is felt (e.g. for three months? six months?) or sustained.

How is a decision made, based on trial information?

This is never easy but initially it is important that enough patients were recruited to give value to the study: 300 are better than 30. The statistics are examined to see whether they reach 'significance' and that should be highlighted in the conclusions or even the initial abstract of the report. It will often say that the 'difference was statistically significant' and quote a 'probability' (p) value – the result of the statistical calculation made.

There may be times when the study did not go on long enough and so the results did not reach statistical significance, or the study recruited enough patients to reach statistical significance in one area but not in another.

It is often difficult to tease out the detail from an article or scientific paper but the bottom line in acute drug treatment for migraine is:

- Is the patient headache-free at 2 hours?
- Is there a sustained pain-free response?
- Does 'rescue' medication have to be taken?
- Are the side effects less than with a placebo?

And, for preventative drugs:

- Is there a reduction in the total number of headache days?
- Is there a greater than 50% reduction in headache days?
- How long did the drug have to be taken for an effect to be seen?
- At what dose did the drug need to be taken for maximum benefit to be achieved?
- Are the side effects less than with a placebo?

As is often the case, there is a trade-off between effectiveness and side effects. Decision-making is never easy, and rarely straightforward. There is no drug out there that will fix all of your headaches all of the time. Hopefully, as more is known and understood about headache symptoms, newer drugs will be developed that work well.

How can I become involved in research?

There are always trials going on somewhere, and the best source of information is probably the headache charities whose websites are listed in Appendix 1.

Alternatively, many of the specialist headache centres around the UK will be involved in research of some sort, although not always drug-based research. Some research uses special types of brain scan to understand more about what happens in the brain; other trials are about understanding more about what effect migraine and other headaches have on your life – impact studies. Other types of research are looking at interventions such as acupuncture or osteopathy to see if they help headache patients.

How are patients selected for trials?

Patients tend to be selected on the basis of their headache diagnosis in the first instance, then on their age and whether they are interested in being involved. You need to be aware that you may not be given any active drug or intervention but will be given the dummy or placebo drug or intervention instead.

There are always strict inclusion and exclusion criteria that depend on the question being asked. If the trial is for acute treatments, you have to be prepared to use only the trial drug for a series of attacks; often patients are selected only if they have never treated their migraine with anything other than simple painkillers; it just depends.

If the trial is for a preventative drug, there are other inclusion and exclusion criteria that apply. For example, the number of headache days each week or month, how many different preventative drugs you have tried in the past and at what doses you tried them, whether you took them for long enough.

How do I know that a new drug is safe to take?

This is always difficult to answer, as newspaper headlines sometimes attest. Drugs will have gone through significant assessment and evaluation before they are given to humans, but all animal and computer models are just that – a model. There is no way to predict exactly what effect a drug will have on the human body until it is administered for the first time.

If you want to become involved in a drug trial, you will be given a lot of information to read, absorb and understand. It is your responsibility to make sure that you clearly do understand and ask all and any questions that need an answer before you are ready to sign the consent form.

In many ways there is no way of knowing a drug is safe until it has been used for many years. Drugs that have been used for decades have been found to be associated with previously unrecognised risks. Sometimes it is about weighing up the balance of potential and theoretical risk against the benefit you get.

If I agree to be involved in a trial and I feel that I am getting worse, can I opt out?

You can opt out at any time. When you do so you will be asked a series of questions so that the researchers doing the trial can understand why: this helps them assess all potential problems associated with the drug or intervention they are investigating.

BOTULINUM TOXIN AND HEADACHE: DOES IT HELP?

Botox is one of those areas where everyone knows someone who feels that it helped them. The evidence, however, is not quite so positive, which is always disappointing, especially with such positive anecdotal experiences.

What is Botox?

Botox is a brand name for botulinum toxin A. Botulinum toxin is a neurotoxin, and is produced by a particular bug (bacterium) called *Clostridium botulinum*, which can cause botulism. Botulism is a condition of paralysis that affects both sides of the body and was thought, in the early 19th century, to be caused by eating spoiled sausage. The Latin for 'black sausage' is botulus, hence botulism.

The toxin was first used to treat spasm in muscles, hence the popularity now with people wanting Botox injections for their facial wrinkles. It is also used to treat muscle problems in a wide range of conditions, including muscle spasm in people who have had a stroke and, more recently, for patients with headache.

Is there any evidence that Botox can help tension-type headache?

Half of the studies done so far have looked at Botox and tension-type headaches. Of the good-quality studies (see above to understand what that means) there was no evidence to support the use of Botox in treating tension-type headache. Of the middle-ranking, not quite so good, studies two said it helped and two said it didn't. It was only the poorest quality studies that found it could help.

Is there any evidence that Botox can help migraine?

As with tension-type headache, one has to reflect on the quality of the studies and again it was only the poorest studies (three) that suggested it could help with migraine symptoms. The better studies gave conflicting reports, one saying it helped and the other saying it did not.

What constitutes a good Botox study?

As I have indicated in the first section of this chapter, there must be enough patients in both the active and the placebo groups. It is crucial that the patients taking part have the correct diagnosis, be it tension-type headache or migraine. Many of the studies on Botox were small, and may well have been too small to show a significant difference between the active and the placebo groups.

With Botox there must be consistency of the injection site among individuals and among study groups. There must also be standardisation of the dose of Botox, and different doses need to be used to see which dose, if any, is effective.

Is Botox safe?

Although Botox is a toxin, it is generally accepted that it is safe at low doses. In the studies that looked at the use of Botox, side effects were reported more commonly in the treatment groups than in the placebo groups.

The sorts of side effects reported included:

- facial weakness
- difficulty swallowing
- disturbed/unusual local sensation
- pain at the injection site
- muscle cramps
- flu-like symptoms
- feeling of weakness of neck muscles
- transient, short-lived weakness of the eyelids or neck, or both
- transient pain in the neck or jaw joint

What about the future and Botox?

There is no doubt that, before a final decision is reached about Botox, we need good studies that look at the different headache types, including migraine, tension-type headache and medication overuse headache, as well as cluster headache.

There must be studies that look at the dose needed to produce benefit and at exactly where those doses should be injected. There also needs to be adequate recording and documentation of side effects in both the treatment and the placebo groups.

INJECTION OF THE GREATER OCCIPITAL NERVE

Nerve 'blocks' have been used to relieve the pain in a variety of situations and medical conditions, including the following:

- pain control during surgery, avoiding the need for a general anaesthetic

- pain control for patients with fractured bones
- neuralgia resulting from local injury or trauma to the nerve
- nerve pain caused by cancer

What is a nerve block?

A nerve block is a way of altering or modifying the response of a nerve so that pain cannot be felt or experienced. It can be done in a variety of ways, including the injection of a local anaesthetic, usually between the site of injury or damage and the spinal cord, thereby altering the pain response.

Another method uses a high radiofrequency signal that causes the nerve to become hot, resulting in damage to the nerve and thus in a permanent break of communication between the nerve, the spinal cord and therefore the brain. Traditionally this was done by heating the nerve to 80°C for 60 to 90 seconds, resulting in the destruction of the nerve. Currently a 'pulsed' method is used with a more gentle process, gradually heating the nerve to 42°C for 10 to 15 minutes, which means that the nerve is not destroyed but the pain response is altered.

In some patients – usually only those with life-threatening or terminal conditions – the nerve might be destroyed by injecting it with a solution designed to kill it.

What is used when doing a nerve block?

Different specialists and different centres use different drugs and drug combinations. Generally, a local anaesthetic is used and this can be combined with a steroid. Studies looking at occipital nerve block have considered both local anaesthetics alone and local anaesthetic combined with steroid.

What can be done to make the nerve block as effective as possible?

Generally speaking, the right balance of local anaesthetic and steroid must be used and has to be injected in the right area to produce the desired nerve block.

Are nerve blocks safe?

In the right hands, yes, they are but remember that no procedure or intervention is totally without risk. There is always the chance that the nerve is missed and no benefit achieved. There is a chance that an infection may develop at the injection site but if appropriate sterile techniques are used this should not occur. If the needle is slightly out of position then other nerves may be affected, but this effect will wear off. If too much drug is used, the effect may be prolonged – often not a bad thing.

What is a greater occipital nerve block?

The greater occipital nerve is shown in Figure 16.1. The nerve is located by the clinician who is doing the block, using specific markers on the scalp, and the area is palpated (felt) to find where there is maximal tenderness – basically where it hurts the most. The skin is cleaned, the needle is inserted and a mix of steroid and local anaesthetic is injected over an area designed to produce an adequate block.

What is the evidence that greater occipital nerve block is effective for headache symptoms?

The evidence, as always, is mixed. Some studies show that it can help some headaches but others are less conclusive. There is no doubt that nerve blocks are very helpful in the management of neuralgia, but the current evidence base is by no means conclusive in relation to headache.

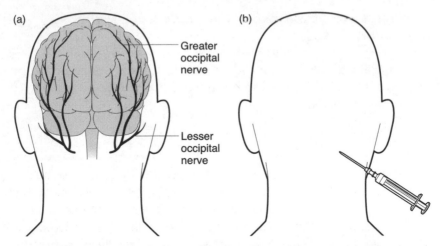

Figure 16.1 (a) The location of the greater and lesser occipital nerves. (b) Injecting into the origin of the greater occipital nerve.

What about the future? Is there a place for nerve blocks in the management of headache patients?

There must be a range of good-quality double-blind placebo-controlled trials looking carefully at the response to occipital nerve blocks in patients with each of the different types of headaches, including migraine, tension-type headache and medication overuse headache as well as cluster headache.

WHAT ABOUT 'HOLES IN THE HEART'? PFO AND MIGRAINE

Of all the things to hit the headlines recently 'hole in the heart' – patent foramen ovale (PFO) – has, in many ways, been the most exciting but also the most controversial. There is no doubt that there is an association between a PFO and migraine. There is also no doubt that closing a large PFO to try to prevent stroke may be appropriate, but

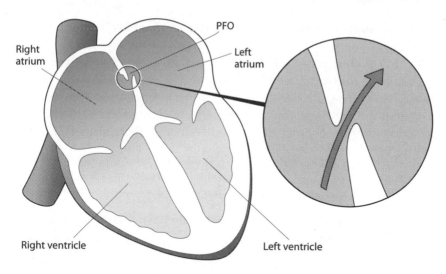

Figure 16.2 A patent foramen ovale (PFO).

the big question is: are the potential risks of surgery worth it in the context of migraine? At the time of writing, the evidence does not support PFO closure, despite the high level of interest and enthusiasm generated by anecdotal evidence.

What actually is a patent foramen ovale?

A foramen ovale is the opening between the two upper chambers of the heart – the atria (singular = atrium) – that allows the blood to circulate oxygen safely and effectively in the fetus (baby) during pregnancy (see Figure 16.2). After the baby is born the foramen ovale closes in 75–85% of cases. If it remains open, it is called 'patent', hence the term patent foramen ovale, or PFO.

The atria normally allow blood to pass from the venous circulation to the ventricles. On the right side this means blood passes from the body to the right ventricle and from there to the lungs, collecting oxygen along the way before passing back to the left atrium, to the left ventricle and from there back to the body.

What conditions might be associated with a PFO?

A PFO has been recognised coincidentally at post-mortem in up to 30% of individuals. Most people with a PFO have no symptoms related to its presence. As patients with specific medical conditions are looked at more closely, the picture seems to change a little, but this is an association; deciding on cause and effect is something else again.

- *Stroke*: In people who have had a stroke under the age of 50 years, between 40 and 60% had a PFO; the larger the PFO the more likely they were to have had a stroke.

- *Divers*: As many as 60% of divers who have had recurrent bouts of decompression sickness ('the bends') have been found to have a PFO.

- *Migraine*: Studies so far have found that 22–57% (higher than the 'control' population) of patients with migraine with aura have a PFO, and 14–21% (similar to the 'control' population) of those with migraine without aura have a PFO.

How can a PFO be diagnosed?

There are a variety of techniques used to diagnose a PFO, including:

- transthoracic echocardiography (TTE, through the chest)

- transoesophageal echocardiography (TEE, through the oesophagus, the tube from the back of your throat to your stomach)

- transcranial Doppler (TCD) imaging (through the base of the skull)

An *echocardiogram* is a way of looking at how the heart is pumping. It uses ultrasound waves to produce a visual display of the heart on a monitor.

A contrast transthoracic echocardiogram was used to screen patients for the MIST (Migraine Intervention with STARFlex Technology) study.

What is the MIST study?

The MIST study was the first to have a placebo, or sham, part to the study. Patients selected for the study had migraine with aura and had failed to respond to two previous preventative drugs. Patients in the placebo group were taken to the catheter lab, anaesthetised and had an incision made so they had no way of knowing whether they had had a device fitted. This was done because it was recognised that the highest quality study was needed to answer the questions relating to PFOs and migraine, and whether PFOs should be closed if found in migraine sufferers.

How can a PFO be closed?

PFOs are closed using any of a variety of devices; the one used in the MIST trial was called STARFlex. This can best be described as a double-layered umbrella that, when opened, can sit either side of the hole and cover it up, hence it is 'closed' (see Figure 16.3).

How does the implant get to where the PFO is in the heart?

A tube (catheter) is inserted into the femoral vein (a vein in the leg) and moved through the venous system to the heart. This is done in a sterile operating theatre under the guidance of echocardiography, which allows the surgeon to see exactly where the catheter is and to make sure it is put into the right place.

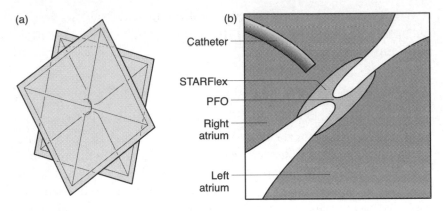

Figure 16.3 (**a**) The STARFlex implant. (**b**) The implant in position, closing the PFO.

What are the risks associated with closing a PFO?

The safety of this sort of procedure depends in large part on the skill of the surgeon. No procedure is without risk but complications on the whole are fortunately rare; they include:

- short-lived heart arrhythmias (irregular heart beats)
- damage to the vein, or bleeding at the site where the catheter is inserted
- damage to the heart muscle
- reaction to medication used during the procedure

In the MIST study the complications in the active group included:

- cardiac tamponade (pressure on the heart from fluid collecting in the sac around it)
- pericardial effusion (fluid collecting in the sac that surrounds the heart)

- retroperitoneal bleed (bleeding within the abdomen)
- atrial fibrillation (an irregular heart beat)
- chest pain

And in the placebo, or sham, group:

- bleeding at the incision site (where the catheter is inserted)
- anaemia
- nose bleed
- brainstem stroke

Will closing a PFO really cure migraine?

The answer to your question is that closing the PFO will not completely 'cure' your migraine. It may reduce the number of headache days you have but so will a variety of other drugs or interventions. Closing a PFO is not without risk and needs to be considered very carefully.

The MIST study showed that there was a 37% reduction in the number of headaches in the intervention group compared with 17% in the placebo group. This suggests that closing the PFO on the basis of the current evidence is no better than current preventative options.

Glossary

Words given in *italic* in the definitions are also defined in this Glossary.

acute in the context of a disease or symptom, severe but of short duration (see also *chronic*)

acute treatment a treatment used to treat the *acute* phase of a symptom or disease process; e.g. a painkiller to treat a headache or back pain (see also *preventative/prophylactic*)

AED anti-epilepsy drug

ataxia an unsteadiness or clumsiness when moving your arms or legs

aura this term is used to describe the symptoms or series of symptoms of an impending attack of either migraine or epilepsy

autosomal dominant an autosomal chromosome is any one of the *chromosomes* that is not a sex chromosome (X or Y); 'dominant' relates to how the chromosome expresses the heritable characteristics

benign a benign headache is one that is not associated with any underlying problem or physical cause; it has no 'harmful' cause. The opposite of *sinister*

biochemical relating to the chemical processes and substances which occur within living organisms, that enable all human cells and organs to function and be healthy – in this instance the brain and nervous system

biofeedback the use of electronic monitoring of a normally automatic bodily function in order to train someone to voluntarily control that function; e.g. using an electromyograph (EMG), muscle contraction can be seen and the individual can learn, by watching the monitor, to relax

BNF, British National Formulary a book that lists the drugs used in the UK to treat medical conditions, grouped according to the diseases they treat. It also indicates the dosages of those drugs as well as side effects, cautions and contraindications

brand name see *proprietary drug*

chromosome a threadlike structure that appears in every living cell, which carries the genetic information in the form of genes

chronic in the context of a disease or symptom, persisting for a long time or constantly recurring (see also *acute*)

class, of drugs in this context relates to a group of drugs of a similar chemical formula, having a similar effect; e.g. beta-blockers, ACE inhibitors, triptans

class effect a group of drugs that have the same properties or effects or side effects or ability to treat a particular condition or disease

CNS central nervous system: the brain and spinal cord (see also *peripheral nervous system*)

compound painkiller/analgesic a painkiller with more than one active ingredient; e.g. co-codamol has paracetamol and codeine in it

cortex in the context of the brain and brain structure: the outer layer, the grey matter that forms the outer part of the brain substance

cranial nerves there are 12 pairs of nerves that arise from the brain itself and not from the spinal cord. Their functions are: I – smell; II – vision; III, IV and VI – eye movements; V – sensation of face, chewing; VII – facial muscles; VIII – hearing and balance; IX – movement of the palate, taste; X – function of the parasympathetic nervous system; XI – some shoulder muscles; XII – tongue movements

criterion (plural = criteria) a symptom (or collection of symptoms) by which a diagnosis may be made

diagnosis the process of identifying the nature of a condition – a headache – by an assessment of the symptoms experienced by the patient during an episode of headache and how that headache develops and evolves over time

diagnostic a symptom that is so distinctive as to lead to the diagnosis of a particular headache

diplopia double vision

dysarthria a condition in which the speech is slurred, and there is difficulty saying words

electroencephalography (EEG) the recording of the electrical activity of the brain

electromyography (EMG) the recording of the electrical activity of muscles

endorphins chemicals (peptides) secreted within the brain and nervous system, the body's natural painkillers

enteric-coated a tablet that is coated in a layer to prevent it from being absorbed before it reaches the intestine

enzyme a biological substance that speeds up chemical reactions

epilepsy an epileptic attack is caused by abnormal electrical activity in the brain and consists of either involuntary movements of the body or loss of consciousness. It can be either inherited or acquired owing to a structural abnormality of the brain (e.g. stroke, tumour or brain damage)

episodic occurring occasionally and at irregular intervals

familial a tendency for diseases or conditions to run in families

fortification spectra visual aura, so called because its zigzag lines resemble a castellated fort

generic drug the scientific name given to a drug (see also *proprietary drug*)

GI glycaemic index – a calculation of how quickly a food is broken down into its constituent parts, specifically looking at glucose, by the digestive system; a high GI food is broken down quickly and a low GI food is broken down more slowly

GP general practitioner

GPwSI a general practitioner (GP) with a special interest – e.g. in headaches

haemorrhagic stroke a stroke that has occurred as a result of a haemorrhage, or bleeding, into the brain

hemianopia blindness of half of a *visual field*

hemisphere one side of the brain; 'hemi' means half

high-impact headache a headache that prevents you from undertaking your normal activities

holistic taking into account the whole person from a social and mental perspective rather than just the medical and disease perspective

hormone a chemical substance that controls certain functions of the body

IHS International Headache Society, a group of individuals and organisations from around the world with an interest in headache

ischaemia lack of blood to a body tissue

ischaemic stroke a stroke that occurs as a result of a loss of blood supply to part of the brain (see also *haemorrhagic stroke*)

lithium a light metal, whose 'salt' is used as a tranquilliser, particularly in dampening mood swings. It is also used in the treatment of *chronic* cluster headache

low-impact headache a headache that does not prevent you from undertaking your normal day-to-day activities

MAOI monoamine oxidase inhibitor, a drug used in the treatment of depression

migraine day a day during which you have migraine, usually counted up over a period of days or weeks to evaluate your response or lack of response to treatment

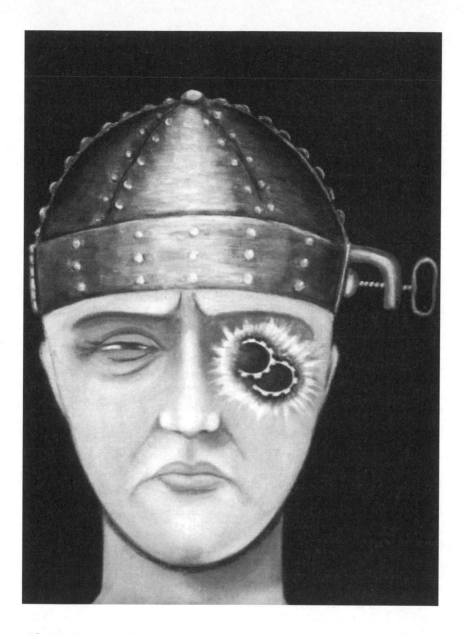

Plate 3 From the Migraine Art collection, reproduced by kind permission of the Migraine Action Association and Boehringer Ingelheim

migraine threshold the point below which a migraine attack becomes inevitable, or above which a migraine attack never occurs

Migraleve a drug available with or without a prescription to treat migraine

MOH medication overuse headache

monosodium glutamate (MSG) a substance used to increase the flavour of foods (found especially in Chinese cuisine)

motor relates to muscular movement or the nerves that stimulate or activate that movement

neuralgia intense intermittent pain that follows the path of a nerve

neurological, neurology the branch of medicine that deals with the anatomy, functions and organic disorders of the nervous system

neurologist a doctor who has undertaken specialist training in *neurology*

neurone a nerve cell

neurophysiology the study of the way the nervous system works

neurotransmitter a chemical substance that is released at the end of a nerve fibre when a nerve impulse arrives and transfers that impulse from one nerve fibre to the next across the gap (*synapse*) between two adjacent nerve cells

oral (dose) taken by mouth, swallowed; usually with water

organic a disease affecting the structure of an organ; this may be a lump or swelling in the skin or a tumour in the brain

paraesthesiae abnormal skin sensations, which include tingling and numbness

pathology the science of the causes and effects of diseases, especially the examination of tissue for *diagnostic* purposes

pathophysiology the disordered physiological process associated with disease or injury

peripheral nervous system the part of the nervous system beyond the brain and spinal cord

phonophobia sensitivity to sound (also referred to as hyperacusia)

photophobia sensitivity to light

physical signs/abnormality 'signs' (or 'findings') are what are discovered as the result of a physical examination, in this case of the nervous system; 'abnormality' relates to the finding that the signs were abnormal

placebo a 'dummy' substance given instead of a drug. Although the help that a placebo has given (particularly for pain) was previously thought to be due to suggestion, recent work suggests that there may be an activation of *endorphins*

preventative/prophylactic a drug used to prevent an attack or condition

Primary Health Care Team (PHCT) health-care professionals involved in patient care, working within the community as opposed to in the hospital. They include the GP, practice nurse, health visitor to name a few

proprietary drug a drug marketed by a specific company and protected by its registered trade mark; also called brand name drug

QOL quality of life

rebound (headache) the recurrence, or bouncing back, of a symptom – in this case a headache – as the result of stopping a medication

recurrence (headache) to occur again, periodically; in this context the headache recurs after a treatment has been given and the effect has worn off

'red flags' signs or symptoms that suggest 'danger' and need urgent assessment and investigation

referred pain pain that is felt to be somewhere in the body other than where it actually occurs

SAH (subarachnoid haemorrhage) a bleed into the fluid-filled space between the arachnoid membrane and the pia mater in the brain

sciatica pain caused by pressure on the sciatic nerve

scotoma a blind spot in the *visual field*

secondary occurring as a result of damage to an organ, in this case the brain, leading to symptoms that are a direct result of that damage

self-help ideas and options for the individual to try to improve their symptoms or situation

sensorimotor involving both *sensory* and *motor* pathways or functions

sensory involving pathways that relate to sensation or the physical senses

serious (headache) significant or worrying symptoms reflecting a risk of disease, such as a brain tumour (see also *structural* and *sinister*)

serotonergic has an effect similar or identical to *serotonin*

serotonin a compound present in blood platelets and serum that acts as a *neurotransmitter* to constrict blood vessels

simple painkiller/analgesic a painkiller such as aspirin, paracetamol or ibuprofen that has only one active ingredient (see also *compound painkiller* and *triptan*)

sinister (headache) potential for something harmful to occur or develop, such as a brain tumour or a *stroke* (see also *serious* and *structural*)

SSRI selective *serotonin* re-uptake inhibitor, an antidepressant

stereotypical persistent repetition, in this case of a set or series of symptoms

stroke a disturbance of the brain due to either blockage or rupture of a blood vessel

structural cause or **abnormality** an abnormality or derangement of the normal structure of an organ, in this instance the brain (see also *serious* and *sinister*)

synapse a junction between two nerve cells, a minute gap across which impulses pass by the movement of a *neurotransmitter*

TAC trigeminal autonomic cephalalgia

TCAD tricyclic antidepressant

temporal arteritis (cranial arteritis) an inflammatory condition of blood vessels, characterised by severe continuous headache; it occurs only in elderly people

TIA transient ischaemic attack, a mini-stroke; a set of symptoms that are relatively short lived and reversible over a few minutes to hours, rather than leaving residual and permanent symptoms

trade name see *proprietary drug*

tricyclics a class of antidepressant drug (so called because their basic chemical structure consists of three rings)

trigeminal nerve the fifth *cranial nerve*; literally 'three twins' because it has three divisions – ophthalmic, maxillary and mandibular, V1, V2 and V3

trigger anything that sets off a particular action, process or situation

triptan an *acute* treatment for migraine, which is migraine specific, that should be taken as the headache starts (see also *simple painkiller* and *compound painkiller*)

TTH tension-type headache

vasoconstriction constriction (narrowing) of a blood vessel

vasodilation expansion (widening) of the diameter of a blood vessel

visual field the area you can see

washout the removal of a material or substance from the body, in this instance a drug

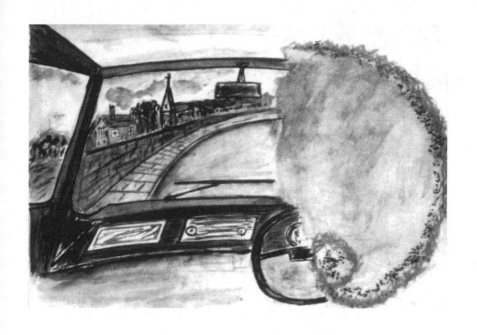

Plate 4 From the Migraine Art collection, reproduced by kind permission
of the Migraine Action Association and Boehringer Ingelheim

Appendix 1
Useful addresses and websites

Migraine Action Association

Founded in 1958, the Migraine Action Association (MAA) is an independent registered charity providing information and support to anyone affected by migraine or disabling primary headaches via its telephone helpline, email and postal information services, two websites (www.migraine.org.uk and www.migraine4kids.org.uk), an extensive range of information leaflets, and a quarterly newsletter, Migraine Action News.

MAA also raises general awareness of migraine and its personal, societal and economic impact, organises local meetings for sufferers, disseminates information on new developments in migraine management, encourages and raises funds for research and supports specialist migraine clinics throughout the UK.

Contact details below.

Migraine Trust

Founded in 1965, the Migraine Trust is a charitable body that distributes information about migraine in the form of a newsletter, a paperback on migraine, a letter-answering service and support of research throughout the UK, and the rest of the world if funds are available. Every two years the Trust organises an International Migraine Symposium at which experts from all over the world gather; the report of their research activities into all aspects of the migraine problem is then published. The money to fund these activities is raised from private donations and fund-raising activities.

Mission statement: 'The Migraine Trust seeks to empower migraine sufferers through information and support whilst educating health professionals and actively funding and disseminating research.'

Contact details below.

**Acupuncture Association
of Chartered Physiotherapists
(AACP)**
Parks Therapy Centre
86 Cambridge Street
St Neots
Cambs PE19 1PJ
Tel: 01480 394739
Fax: 0870 0519230
Website: www.aacp.uk.com
*The regulatory body of physio-
therapists who also practise
acupuncture.*

Alexander Technique
see Society of Teachers of the
Alexander Technique

Aromatherapy Consortium
PO Box 6522
Desborough
Kettering
Northants NN14 2YX
Tel/Fax: 0870 774 3477
(10 a.m.–2 p.m., Mon–Fri)
Website:
www.aromatherapy-regulation.org.uk
*Has a directory of therapists qualified
to national standards.*

**Body Control Pilates
(Association of Pilates Teachers)**
6 Langley Street
London WC2H 9JA
Tel: 020 7379 3734
Fax: 020 7379 7551
Website: www.bodycontrol.co.uk
*Promotes a wider understanding of
Pilates and its benefits for body and
mind.*

**British Acupuncture Council
(BAcC)**
63 Jeddo Road
London W12 9HQ
Tel: 020 8735 0400
Fax: 020 8735 0404
Website: www.acupuncture.org.uk
*Professional body offering lists of
qualified acupuncture therapists.*

**British Association for
the Study of Headache
(BASH: UK)**
Membership enquiries:
Professor Peter Goadsby
University Department of Clinical
Neurology
Institute of Neurology
Queen Square
London WC1N 3BG
Website: www.bash.org.uk
*Member of the IHS; aims to relieve
those affected by headaches.
Membership open to all health-care
professionals interested in headache.*

British Chiropractic Association
59 Castle Street
Reading
Berks RG1 7SN
Tel: 0118 950 5950
Fax: 0118 958 8946
Website: www.chiropractic-uk.co.uk
Professional body promoting high standards in chiropractic in the UK.

British Complementary Medicine Association
PO Box 5122
Bournemouth BH8 0WG
Tel : 0845 345 5977
Website: www.bcma.co.uk
Ensures high-quality standards within the industry.

British Holistic Medical Association
PO Box 371
Bridgwater
Somerset TA6 9BG
Tel: 01278 722000
Website: www.bhma.org
Educating health-care professionals and members of the general public in the principles and practice of holistic medicine. '

British Homeopathic Association
incorporating the
Homeopathic Trust
Hahnemann House
29 Park Street West
Luton LU1 3BE
Tel: 0870 444 3950
Fax: 0870 444 3960
Website: www.trusthomeopathy.org
Professional body offering lists of qualified homoeopathic practitioners.

British Hypnotherapy Association
67 Upper Berkley Street
London W1H 7QX
Tel: 020 7723 4443
Website: www.hypnotherapy-association.org
Maintains a list of practitioners trained to the Association's standards.

British Medical Acupuncture Society
The Administrator, BMAS
3 Winnington Court
Northwich
Cheshire CW8 1AQ
Tel: 01606 786782
Fax: 01606 786783
Website: www.medical-acupuncture.co.uk
Provides a comprehensive list of trained acupuncture practitioners in the UK.

British Osteopathic Association
Langham House West
Mill Street
Luton
Beds LU1 2NA
Tel: 01582 488455
Fax: 01582 481533
Website: www.osteopathy.org
Professional organisation of osteopaths in the UK; provides search facility to locate osteopaths in the UK.

British Pain Society
21 Portland Place
London W1B 1PY
Tel: 020 7631 8870
Fax: 020 7323 2015
Website: www.britishpainsociety.org
Multidisciplinary organisation in the UK in the field of pain; provides information for people with pain, including a list of UK-based patient organisations.

British Psychological Society
St Andrews House
48 Princess Road East
Leicester LE1 7DR
Tel: 0116 254 9568
Fax: 0116 247 0787
Website: www.bps.org.uk
To find a hypnotherapist near you.

British Reflexology Association
Monk's Orchard
Whitbourne
Worcester WR6 5RB
Tel: 01886 821207
Fax: 01886 822017
Website: www.britreflex.co.uk
For a list of reflexology practitioners world wide.

British Tinnitus Association
Ground Floor, Unit 5
Acorn Business Park
Woodseats Close
Sheffield S8 0TB
Tel: 0800 018 0527
Fax: 0114 258 2279
Website: www.tinnitus.org.uk
Provides support, advice and information about tinnitus.

British Wheel of Yoga
25 Jermyn Street
Sleaford
Lincolnshire NG34 7RU
Tel: 01529 306851
Fax: 01529 303233
Website: www.bwy.org.uk
Registered charity that promotes yoga classes to the general public.

General Chiropractic Council
44 Wicklow Street
London WC1X 9HL
Tel: 020 7713 5155
Fax: 020 7713 5844
Website: www.gcc-uk.org
The regulatory body for chiropractors in the UK. Has a list of registered therapists in the UK.

General Hypnotherapy Register
PO Box 204
Lymington SO41 6WP
Tel/Fax: 01590 683770
Website: www.general-hypnotherapy-register.com
The administrative agency for the General Hypnotherapy Standards Agency. Provides a list of registered therapists in the UK.

General Osteopathic Council
Osteopathy House
176 Tower Bridge Road
London SE1 3LU
Tel: 020 7357 6655
Fax: 020 7357 0011
Website: www.osteopathy.org.uk
Regulatory body that offers information to the public and lists of accredited osteopaths.

Headache UK
55–56 Russell Square
London WC1B 4HP
Tel: 020 7436 1336/2880
Fax: 020 7436 2880
Website: www.headacheuk.org
An alliance for people with headaches.

Health & Safety Executive
Rose Court
2 Southwark Bridge
London SE1 9HS
Website: www.hse.gov.uk
To order publications:
01787 881165
Responsible for health and safety regulation in Great Britain under the aegis of the Health and Safety Commission.

Institute for Complementary Medicine
PO Box 194
London SE16 1QZ
Tel: 020 7237 5165
Fax: 020 7237 5175
Website: www.l-c-m.org.uk
Administers the British Register of Complementary Practitioners (BRCP). Provides information on complementary medicine.

**International Federation
of Aromatherapists**
61–63 Churchfield Road
London W3 6AY
Tel: 020 8992 9605
Fax: 020 8992 7983
Website: www.ifaroma.org
*Send a cheque for £2.50 with an A5
s.a.e. for a list of therapists nationwide.*

**McTimoney Chiropractic
Association**
Crowmarsh Gifford
Wallingford OX10 8DJ
Tel: 01491 829211
Fax: 01491 829492
Website: www.mctimoney-chiropractic.org
*Send a cheque or postal order for
£1.50 and a 50p stamp for a list of
practitioners.*

**Massage Therapy Institute
of Great Britain**
Clare Maxwell-Hudson
School of Massage
Lower Ground Floor
20 Enford Street
London W1H 1DG
Tel: 020 7724 7198
Website: www.cmhmassage.co.uk
*Send an s.a.e. for information and a
list of therapists in your area.*

Meningitis Research Foundation
Midland Way
Thornbury
Bristol BS35 2BS
Helpline: 0808 800 3344 (24 hours)
Tel: 01454 281811
Fax: 01454 281094
Website: www.meningitis.org
*A support organisation that funds
research to prevent meningitis and
septicaemia, improve survival rates
and promote education and awareness.*

Meningitis Trust
Fern House
Bath Road
Stroud
Gloucestershire GL5 3TJ
Helpline: 0845 6000 800 (24-hours)
Tel: 01453 768 000
Fax: 01453 768001
Website: www.meningitis-trust.org
*Works toward a world free from
meningitis; the helpline is led by
specially trained nurses.*

Migraine Action Association
(*formerly* **British Migraine Association**)
Unit 6
Oakley Hay Lodge Business Park
Great Folds Road
Great Oakley
Northants NN18 9AS
Tel: 01536 461 333
Fax: 01536 461 444
Website: www.migraine.org.uk
Provides information and support for people with migraine and their families. Migraine Awareness Week is held during the first week of September.
See also the information in the box at the beginning of this appendix.

Migraine in Primary Care Advisors (MiPCA)
Website: www.mipca.org.uk
An independent charity of health-care professionals working through research and education to set standards for the care of headache sufferers.

Migraine Trust
2nd Floor
55–56 Russell Square
London WC1B 4HP
Tel: 020 7436 1336
Fax: 020 7436 2880
Website: www.migrainetrust.org
Provides information and support to migraine sufferers.
See also the information in the box at the beginning of this appendix.

NHS Direct
Tel: 0845 4647
Textphone: 0845 606 4647
Website: www.nhsdirect.nhs.uk
A 24-hour helpline offering confidential healthcare advice, information and referral service 365 days of the year.

NHS Healthpoint
Tel: 0800 66 55 44
(freephone 9 a.m.–5 p.m.)
Health information service funded by the NHS.

NHS24
Tel: 08454 24 24 24
Textphone: 18001 08454 24 24 24
Website: www.nhs24.com
Provides confidential telephone health advice and information service for people in Scotland.

National Council of Hypnotherapy
PO Box 421
Charwelton
Daventry NN11 1AS
Tel: 0800 952 0545
Website: www.hypnotherapists.org.uk
Primarily for health-care professionals; publishes Understanding and Managing Pain *for patients and has a register of hypnotherapists in the UK.*

**National Institute
of Medical Herbalists**
Elm House
54 Mary Arches Street
Exeter EX4 3BA
Tel: 01392 426022
Fax: 01392 498963
Website: www.nimh.org.uk
*Pofessional body representing herbal
medicine practitioners; promotes the
benefits of herbal medicine.*

**OUCH (UK)
Organisation for
the Understanding of
Cluster Headaches (UK)**
c/o Errington Langer and Pinner
Pyramid House
956 High Road
London N12 9RX
Helpline: 0161 272 1702
Website: www.clusterheadache.org
*Provides support, information and
advice on coping with cluster
headaches.*

**Over-Count
Drugs Information Agency**
9 Croft Road
Bankend
Dumfries DG1 4RW
Tel: 01387 770404 (11 a.m.–4 p.m.
Mon–Sat + 6–10 p.m. Tues)
Website: www.over-count.org.uk
*Independent advice and information
about over-the-counter,
non-prescription medicines.*

Pain Concern
PO Box 13256
Haddington EH41 4YD
Tel: 01620 822572
Website: www.painconcern.org.uk
*Run by chronic pain sufferers, it
provides information and support to
pain sufferers and their families.*

Pilates
see **Body Control Pilates**

**Register of
Chinese Herbal Medicine**
Office 5, 1 Exeter Street
Norwich NR2 4QB
Tel: 01603 623994
Fax: 01603 667557
Website: www.rchm.co.uk
*Send a cheque or postal order for £2
with an A5 sae for a list of qualified
practitioners in your area.*

Reiki Association
2 Spa Terrace
Fenay Bridge
Huddersfield HD8 0BD
Tel/Fax: 0901 8800 009
Website: www.reikiassociation.org.uk
*Association fostering the practice of
Reiki.*

**Scottish Massage Therapists'
Organisation**
70 Lochside Road
Aberdeen AB23 8QW
Tel/Fax: 01224 822960
Website: www.scotmass.co.uk
*Contains a Register of massage
therapists*

Society of Homeopaths
11 Brookfield
Duncan Close
Moulton Park
Northampton NN3 6WL
Tel: 0845 450 6611
Fax: 0845 450 6622
Website: www.homeopathy-soh.com
*Organisation of professional
homeopaths.*

**Society of Teachers of the
Alexander Technique (STAT)**
1st Floor, Linton House
39–51 Highgate Road
London NW5 1RS
Helpline: 0845 230 7828
Tel: 020 7284 3338
Fax: 020 7482 5435
Website: www.stat.org.uk
*Offers general information and lists of
teachers of the Alexander Technique in
the UK and world-wide, and
recommended training schools.*

Stroke Association
240 City Road
London EC1V 2PR
Helpline: 0845 30 33 100
Tel: 020 7566 0300
Fax: 020 7490 2686
Website: www.stroke.org.uk
*Helps stroke patients and their
families, providing information
services and welfare grants. Also funds
research.*

**Trigeminal Neuralgia
Association UK**
PO Box 413
Bromley
Kent BR2 9XS
Tel: 020 8462 9122 (Head Office)
Website: www.tna.org.uk
*Provides information and offers
support to members, and raises
awareness of TN among medical
professionals as well as the general
public.*

**World Headache Alliances
(WHA: International)**
Website: www.w-h-a.org
*An alliance that shares information
among headache organisations and
works to increase the awareness and
understanding of headache.*

Index

Page numbers in *italics* indicate illustrations and tables; italic *g* after a page number indicates an entry in the Glossary.

internet, researching on the 284–5
irritability 144
ischaemic strokes 28, 271, 304*g*
   and HRT 276–7
   see also transient ischaemic
      attacks
itraconazole *180*

ketoconazole *180*

levetiracetam 200, 202, 273
light, sensitivity to/photophobia 11,
   16, 33, *88*, 150
lighting conditions 14, 80, 81, 92,
   242
lights, seeing *see* auras; flashing
   lights
Linde Gas UK (oxygen suppliers)
   188
lithium 206, 208, 209, 304*g*
LNG-IUS (levonorgestrel intra-
   uterine system) coil 279, 282

magnesium 121
MAOIs (monoamine oxidase
   inhibitors) *181*, 304*g*
massage therapies 112–15, 210,
   211
Maxolon 168
meal patterns 80, 82, 84, 85, 90,
   91, 156
   of children 240
meat, red (as trigger) 89
medication
   acute 166–74; *see also* triptans
   over-the-counter 99–101
   preventative *see* preventative
      treatments

and safety 290–1
   see also medication overuse
      headaches
medication overuse headaches
   (MOHs) 3, 34, *34*, 35–6, 38–9,
   125–6, 160, 191, 210,
   212–13
   in children 235, 236
   duration and frequency 28, 32,
      37, 41
   and stopping painkillers 35, 38,
      39–43, 164–5, 213–23
   see also triptans
meditation 117, 118
meningeal membranes *69*, 70
meningitis 70–1
menopausal migraines 9–10, 24,
   75, 274–6
   and HRT 276–9
menstrual cycle 84, 254–5
menstrual migraines (MM) 12,
   174, 255–7
   diet and lifestyle changes 263,
      264
   hormone treatments 258–9
menstrually associated migraine
   (MAM) 12, 257–8
methysergide *180*, *181*
metoclopramide 167, 168, 169,
   172, 185, 226, 227, 262, 270
metoprolol 197
midwives, community 135–6
migraine 5, 6
   classical 12–13
   common 12–13
   duration of attacks 15, 23, 28
   frequency of attacks 18, 23
   phases 15, *16*, 24, *88*

Have you found *Migraine and other Headaches: Answers at your fingertips* useful and practical? If so, you may be interested in other books from Class Publishing.

HIGH BLOOD PRESSURE
Answers at your fingertips   £14.99

Dr Julian Tudor Hart with Dr Tom Fahey

The authors use all their years of experience as blood pressure experts
to answer your questions on high blood pressure, in order to give you the information you need to bring your blood pressure down – and keep it down.

> *'Readable and comprehensive information.'*
>
> Dr Sylvia McLaughlan,
> former Director General,
> The Stroke Association

THE BACK PAIN BOOK   £17.99

Mike Hage

Nearly two-thirds of adults in the UK have had experience of back pain. Now there's hope – and help – for the sufferer. Instead of addressing specific medical diagnoses, the book offers guidance on how to use posture and movement to ease, relieve and prevent back pain.

> *'The book is the most comprehensive book I have come across as a self-help guide to back problems.'*
>
> Richard Perry, London

STROKE
Answers at your fingertips   £17.99

Dr Anthony Rudd, Penny Irwin and Bridget Penhale

This essential guidebook tells you all about strokes and, most importantly, how to recover from them.

As well as providing clear explanations of the medical processes, tests and treatments, the book is full of practical advice, including recuperation plans. You will find it inspiring.

> *'An excellent and long overdue book.'*
>
> Donal O'Kelly, Director,
> Different Strokes

MENOPAUSE
Answers at your fingertips   £17.99

Dr Heather Currie

The average age of the menopause is 51 years, but it can occur much earlier or later. The symptoms vary widely in their severity, and can include hot flushes, night sweats, palpitations, insomnia, joint pain and headaches. Women are at greater risk of osteoporosis after the menopause.

This invaluable guide answers hundreds of questions from women approaching or experiencing the menopause, and provides positive, practical advice on a range of issues.

DIABETES
Answers at your fingertips   £14.99

Professor Peter Sönksen, Dr Charles Fox and Sue Judd

This is an invaluable reference guide for people with diabetes, which offers practical advice on every aspect of living with the condition, giving you the knowledge and reassurance you need to deal confidently with your diabetes.

> *'I have no hesitation in commending this book.'*
>
> Sir Steve Redgrave CBE,
> Vice President, Diabetes UK

BEATING DEPRESSION   £17.99

Dr Stefan Cembrowicz and Dr Dorcas Kingham

Depression is one of most common illnesses in the world – affecting up to one in four people at some time in their lives. Beating Depression shows sufferers and their families that they are not alone, and offers tried and tested techniques for overcoming depression.

> *'This is a very good, comprehensive book that is easy to use and follow.'*
>
> Amelia Mustapha,
> The Depression Alliance

PRIORITY ORDER FORM

Cut out or photocopy this form and send it (post free in the UK) to:

Class Publishing   **Tel: 01256 302 699**
FREEPOST 16705   **Fax: 01256 812 558**
Macmillan Distribution
Basingstoke RG21 6ZZ

Please send me urgently   *Post included*
(tick below)   *price per copy (UK only)*

☐ **Migraine and other Headaches – Answers at your fingertips**
  (ISBN 1 85959 149 2)   £17.99

☐ **High Blood Pressure – Answers at your fingertips** (ISBN 1 85959 090 X)   £17.99

☐ **The Back Pain Book** (ISBN 1 85959 124 8)   £20.99

☐ **Stroke – Answers at your fingertips** (ISBN 1 85959 113 2)   £20.99

☐ **Menopause – Answers at your fingertips** (ISBN 1 85959 155 8)   £20.99

☐ **Diabetes – Answers at your fingertips** (ISBN 1 85959 087 X)   £17.99

☐ **Beating Depression** (ISBN 1 85959 150 7)   £20.99)

                                              TOTAL _____

Easy ways to pay

Cheque: I enclose a cheque payable to Class Publishing for £ _____

Credit card: Please debit my   Mastercard ☐ Visa ☐ Amex ☐ Switch

Number _____ Expiry date _____

Name _____

My address for delivery is _____

_____

Town _____ County _____ Postcode _____

Telephone number (*in case of query*) _____

Credit card billing address if different from above _____

_____

Town _____ County _____ Postcode _____

Class Publishing's guarantee: remember that if, for any reason, you are not satisfied with these books, we will refund all your money, without any questions asked. Prices and VAT rates may be altered for reasons beyond our control.